RED HOT TANTRA

RED HOT TANTRA

Erotic Secrets of Red Tantra for Intimate, Soul-to-Soul Sex and Ecstatic, Enlightened Orgasms

DAVID A. RAMSDALE
AND CYNTHIA W. GENTRY

FAIR WINDS
PRESS
GLOUCESTER, MASSACHUSETTS

First published in the USA in 2004 by
Fair Winds Press
33 Commercial Street
Gloucester, MA 01930

08 07 06 05 04 1 2 3 4 5

ISBN 1-59233-051-7

Library of Congress Cataloging-in-Publication Data available

Cover design by Mary Ann Smith
Book design by Laura Herrmann Design

Printed and bound in Canada

To my parents, for their loving support and spiritual example, and to Divine Mother, for making all this possible.
—David A. Ramsdale, M.A.

To Nima, my muse.
—Cynthia W. Gentry

TABLE OF CONTENTS

CHAPTER FOUR 117

TANTRIC TOUCHING

CHAPTER FIVE 157

TANTRIC SEEING

CHAPTER ONE

What is Red Tantra?

What Is Red Tantra?

Tantra, like sandalwood incense and sitar music, is an Indian import. According to eminent yoga scholar Georg Feuerstein, Ph.D., the type of tantra popular today originated in medieval India around A.D. 1000. This tradition, the source for most of the tantra books and teachings, I call "white tantra."

The complement to white tantra is red tantra. White tantra is the masculine version of the tradition. Red tantra is the feminine form. Some sources explain that these labels came into use because semen is white and menstrual blood is red.

Red tantra is based on the sexual practices of the ancient, even neolithic, goddess traditions. This type of tantra, the most ancient tantra of all, is the mother of white tantra. This red tantra tradition predates the white tantra of India by many thousands of years.

Worship of the mother goddess has been traced back ten thousand years to the Indus Valley in what is now called India. There, a great civilization flourished that archeologists call the Harappa.

Based on the abundance of earth goddess figurines and other archeological evidence in what is now known as Europe and the

Near East, ten thousand years ago the great mother goddess ruled there as well.

In fact, versions of tantra can be found in most cultures in the world. There is Arabic tantra, Hawaiian tantra, Native American tantra, Norse tantra and so forth.

My research indicates that all of these modern variations evolved from a great, tantric mother goddess tradition that was the dominant spiritual movement on the planet long before writing was invented. Tantra was the first religion!

Tantra in the west is now so completely dominated by white tantra that few people, even tantrikas, those who have made tantra an important part of their spiritual path, know about the red tantra alternative.

As a result, there is a gap between playful, sensual, total let-go sex—making love the natural way—and the widely published white tantra ideals of sublimating and controlling sexual energy. Women who are intuitively guided to embrace the lush physicality of a totally uninhibited sexual orgasm may conclude they don't have a place in tantra.

Many white tantra teachers tell female students to deny, suppress or manipulate the natural sexual orgasm. They often advise them to "rise above" their genital sexual climax and achieve some kind of internal energy orgasm. The theory is that it will be vastly superior. The irony is that the one teaching these half-truths is probably a woman.

In contrast, red tantra teaches the exact opposite: The woman's spiritually ideal orgasm is a natural, sensual, total let-go sexual orgasm. Red tantra agrees with the view that a woman is empowered by fully claiming her sexual pleasure.

WHITE TANTRA TECHNOLOGY

Why would white tantra tell a woman to change what is natural for her? What could possibly be wrong with the orgasm, female or male?

Modern society credits man with the dominant sex drive. White tantric and taoist scriptures, however, assert that the woman's capacity for sexual pleasure and orgasm far exceeds that of the man. Some of these ancient sex treatises state that she has nine times the natural erotic talent of a man!

Whether this is true or not, it does say something about the beliefs held by men at that time. My theory is that white tantra was developed by men because they could not sexually compete with women. Specifically, they could not match the known female capacity to achieve wave after wave of internally generated, self-sustaining orgasmic pleasure.

Understandably, these men set out to learn from women in the hopes of duplicating this extraordinary orgasmic capacity within their own male bodies. To a large extent, they succeeded. This male-oriented technology is a complete system for manipulating the internal forces into an ecstatic energy crisis using concentration, exercises, postures, and breath control.

The texts of Hindu and Buddhist white tantra are obsessed with semen retention and achieving an internal orgasm without ejaculation. The anatomy it follows is exclusively male. Some texts even go so far as to advise the tantric or taoist yogi to regard the female as a clever, seductive adversary, an insatiable she-vampire on a secret mission to steal their life-force by sucking out their semen.

For the last twenty years, women have been coming to me for counseling and telling me that white tantra does not feel natural to them. Why should it? The white tantra methods were designed by monks for monks.

In ancient days, the women were the tantric mentors, not the men. As society changed, women realized that their knowledge was about to be lost. They chose to train men in their place rather than lose everything. Over time, as the grip of patriarchal power and the suppression of sexual freedom spread to global domination, it was forgotten that women have their own tantra, the red tantra that mothers used to teach their daughters.

As women lost their natural, goddess-based tantric knowledge and power, they forgot how to transmit spiritual energy through sex as a conscious, sacred art. The sacred temple practices were lobotomized by patriarchal domination into the profane prostitution business of today.

Medieval tantra, the venerable father of modern white tantra, is a powerful, majestic, effective spiritual system. Its discoveries regarding the chakras (energy centers), kundalini (the liberating goddess energy in the body), and sexual energy are remarkable. It deserves deep respect and serious study.

However, the erroneous belief that white tantra is the only tantra has led to an imbalance. Sensitive, caring individuals and couples struggle for years to overcome its artificial approach to lovemaking, often without success. Many, if not most of those who turn to white tantra for fulfillment retreat in confusion, more dissatisfied than ever. After all, tantra is meant to feel like a natural experience, not a man and woman playing monk and nun for a day.

THE TEMPLE DEVADASI TRADITION

Archeological and historical evidence point to an unbroken tradition of sacred sexual worship based on the mother goddess religion. This was the goddess tradition the biblical Hebrews fought as Ashtoreth or Asherah (probably the fertility goddess Astarte, whose erotic practices prospered in their new home of Canaan). This same tradition thrived in rural India until the late nineteenth century as the sacred spiritual path of the devadasi, the holy temple prostitute.

The word prostitute is misleading. Prostitution is what survived the devastation of the once revered devadasi tradition. The word devadasi literally translates to "female slave of the divine."

In the heyday of the devadasi, the divine had not yet become male. At best, he was a temporary, dispensable consort, a kind of summer fling. The divine the devadasis served was the supreme, primal female—goddess, mother, sister, daughter, lover, friend—and even more, the earth, sky and infinite universe itself. The surefire sign that this great goddess of life and love abundant had possessed a woman's body was uniquely joyful and elegantly obvious—she had an orgasm.

This respected position was passed from mother to daughter. For many thousands of years, this role of devadasi was looked upon with approval by civilization. The temples where the priestesses lived, farmed, tended livestock and raised their children, the offspring from unions with temple worshippers, functioned as spiritual centers for men as well as women.

When a man went to the temple to have sex with a devadasi, he believed that he was experiencing union with the goddess herself. The tradition taught that the goddess descended into the sanctified woman and literally took her over during their union. Through the sensual miracle of the sweet grace of the goddess, he was able to actually experience union with the divine. Imagine if churches and synagogues were allowed to offer sacred prostitution with their other services!

For many thousands of years, this down-to-earth system worked smoothly.

Some say invading nomads destroyed it. Others say the invention of writing overstimulated the left brain, resulting in alienation from the goddess and her practices as well as nature itself. Whatever the cause, there is no doubt that, at one time, the religion of the mother goddess and her worship via sacred sex in her temples reigned supreme in the world.

THE ENLIGHTENED VAGINA

There is a tantric text that is a source of controversy in the Buddhist world, though few outside of Buddhism know about it.

The text in Sanskrit, said to be the authenticated words of the Buddha, reads "Buddhatvam Yosityonisamasritam."

In English, this respected tantric scripture quotes the Buddha making the astonishing assertion that "Enlightenment resides in the sexual parts of women."

Buddhism has made enormous efforts from its early beginnings to insure the reliability of its texts. Monk scholars have tried to explain away this embarrassing assertion by the Buddha as merely symbolic. However, this same view is repeated in sacred texts of the tantric Kashmir Shaivite tradition of northern India and other little-known sources, including secret red tantra oral teachings and certain extremely rare Chinese Buddhist texts.

This controversial view, made public by the fearless Buddha, teaches that when a woman is in a state of sexual orgasm she is actually experiencing, and effortlessly transmitting or radiating, a state of enlightenment. The implication, though the Buddha does not actually come out and say it, is that a woman does not need a man in order to have her ultimate sexospiritual experience, the orgasm of nirvana. However, if a man is at the right place at the right time, then he may benefit.

The Buddha's statement can also be interpreted as saying that the key is simply in the sexual union itself, in the physical intimacy of penis and vagina (as in the well-known phrase "diamond in the lotus"). In this view, neither partner needs to orgasm for female transmission and male reception to take place.

I believe both views are correct. I suspect that a woman's mystical transmission is intensified, gathered, and focused by her orgasm. Whether or not orgasms take place, the cervix is, in my opinion, the gateway for her spiritual energy. Swami Satyananda, a tantric master in India, confirmed this for me when he identified the cervix as the center of kundalini in a woman's body.

Kundalini, the mystical sex force within the human body, is the most likely source for such a transformational force. The late Swami Muktananda, a kundalini master, was renowned for his "shaktipat," his ability to transmit shakti. For many, his touch or glance precipitated an extraordinary spiritual experience.

Shakti, of course, is a name for the goddess energy. Who, then, apart from masters such as Swami Muktananda, would be better qualified to give shaktipat than a woman? I believe that the first form of shaktipat on the planet took place as a sexually transmitted spiritual blessing. Temple devadasis routinely provided sexual shaktipat in sacred ceremonies to men everywhere, promoting widespread harmony and happiness.

The ancient tantric authorities place the epicenter of female orgasmic nirvana at what we call the cervix. They assign the g-spot a medium intensity value. They recognize the clitoris as well, but associate it with the most superficial level of stimulation and release. In fact, some contemporary women are reporting prolonged, uniquely spiritual climaxes from direct cervical stimulation alone.

Apparently, these tantric masters recommended a symphonic interweaving of clitoral and g-spot stimulation. The deep g-spot arousal, in turn, tends to awaken the cervical energy center. An erotic musical chord results, with beautiful, sustained vibrations, as clitoris, g-spot and cervix each sound a unique note.

What if direct stimulation of the cervix is pleasurable? Then red tantra certainly recommends a complete exploration of that experience. Please refer to Red Hot Resources in the back.

However, many women find that direct cervical stimulation yields no response. Some even find it painful. There is no evidence that direct stimulation is needed for tantra. I don't want cervical orgasm to be perceived as some kind of new performance pressure!

In the goddess age, women may have enjoyed the full orgasmic spectrum. Perhaps temple priestesses were, in part, chosen for their orgasmic gifts. Possibly they had many ways to assess a woman's capacity to transmit goddess energy.

Echoing certain modern Taoist teachings, the ancient red tantra asserts that the woman experiences "an orgasm of emptiness." When her ego disappears, nirvana appears.

At the peak of her maximum orgasm in which she surrenders totally to her own physical pleasure, she will disappear. She will vanish. She will be gone, gone, gone beyond gone. This is the red tantra teaching for her. This is her direct taste of nirvana.

Some white tantra texts instruct the man to suck this energetic goddess nirvana nectar in through the opening at the tip of his penis and into his body during intercourse. This practice led to bizarre distortions, including a form of energy vampirism still practiced by certain tantric and taoist sects.

How is she to achieve this maximum orgasm? The same way she achieves anything else of value in her life: practice, practice, practice!

Exposure to eastern thought, such as the ideas in this book, is helpful. Then she may recognize that she has just "seen her own true nature." She has entered into the void, she has disappeared, and she has returned. Through red tantra, she has received a revelation of what some people spend many years struggling to experience and never get—a direct, experiential taste of the void, nirvana, the no-self, the ground of being, the universal self, cosmic consciousness.

In red tantra, the orgasm is not denied, suppressed or manipulated. Instead, it is fully experienced. When the woman orgasmed, this was a sign that the goddess was pleased. When the goddess was pleased, then life would be good.

This was the attitude of the neolithic hunters and gatherers and of the early agricultural societies. Thus began the red tantra tradition, handed down woman to woman through the centuries. Though a twisted travesty of the truth, the biblical story of Adam and Eve, did get one thing right: The woman did start it all. She, the sweet fruit of love, created red tantra in those first, unforgettable sacred sexual communions with the goddess in ages lost.

THE GRACE OF THE GODDESS TODAY

This "vaginal nirvana" theory suggests that the sacred meetings with the female representative of the goddess in her temple were precisely that. During intercourse or other sexual acts, the devadasi achieved a nirvana-like state, simultaneously receiving and giving the spiritual gifts of the goddess. The worshipful male, his mind humbled and receptive to the energetic touch of the goddess, may have then experienced true transcendental sex via the grace of the devadasi's ecstatic transmission.

In the early 1970s, at the age of twenty-two, I received just such a transmission and initiation from a female tantric master in Mendocino, California. She lived like a gypsy, splitting her time between the silence of the mountains and the homes of those who recognized her mastery. She was about twice my age.

I do not know if she had a cervical orgasm, as we did not talk about the experience afterwards. I was on top. She lifted her legs up over her shoulders, so that her feet were near her ears. It was a tantric sexual application of a well-known hatha yoga position called "the plow pose" (halasana). I suspect that she knew that this position would enable me to achieve maximum penetration and get as close to her cervix as I could.

I still remember that moment when she swung her legs up and back. I remember being astonished by her flexibility. Then, effortlessly, I slipped more deeply into her than I had thought possible.

Within minutes after that, spontaneously, without any instruction from her other than the magnetic beauty of her presence, the rhythmic power of her breathing, and the amazing compassion in her eyes, I felt my identity dissolve into an ocean of supremely peaceful, blissful white light. This profound ego-death experience, which some would call an experience of enlightenment, was the turning point that led to my lifelong dedication to tantra.

Since this was the 1970s, I think it is important to mention that she and I were not on drugs of any kind. In fact, abstinence was a prerequisite of my student-teacher relationship with her. She lived on wildflowers, herbs, and other vegetarian gifts of the earth. Her lean, lithe, tanned body was her tantric temple.

THE MALE TRANSCENDENTAL ORGASM

Since white tantra was designed by men for men to expand male orgasmic potential and attain sexomystical experiences, certainly a man should familiarize himself with its teachings and tenets. There are many good books available.

However, many men, thinking that the internal, psychotechnological energy orgasm of white tantra is the only true tantric orgasm, become rigid and imbalanced. I have encountered many such highly spiritual, deeply sincere and energetically frozen tantric males in my role as a teacher.

I began working with kundalini energy and the white tantric energy orgasm as a teenager. I have had excellent teachers. I practiced the methods for a decade with delicious results. In fact, I got so good at achieving instant internal sexual bliss that I was able to demonstrate the energy orgasm live and on cue for the Playboy Channel!

I have now gone full circle in my tantric life journey. I now believe that the natural "thunderbolt" orgasm of red tantra, accompanied by ejaculation, is nature's antidote to this stuck, repressed condition. The conventional ejaculation orgasm relieves and releases aggressive male tension. This same orgasm, when approached from a red-tantric understanding, is a profound experience that transforms aggressive male tendencies into spiritual surrender and awakening.

While it is impressive that a man can achieve the female extended orgasm, what is the point? If he looks to nature for guidance, he will see that activities of the earth and sky are very different yet complementary. For the average man who seeks a more spiritual orgasm, nature shows the way.

A river flows and flows merrily, seemingly forever. It is accepted as it is. The thunderbolt strikes the earth with sudden, loud, aggressive brilliance and then is gone. It, too, is accepted as it is. No one says "The thunderbolt is over much too quickly. It should be like a river and continue thundering and flashing and striking the earth for a very long time without stopping."

While there is nothing wrong with achieving the woman's orgasm in a man's body, it misses the mark. There is a natural male orgasm that is the polar opposite of and energetic complement to the female orgasm. As a man achieves greater depths of physical, emotional, and mental surrender during ejaculation orgasm, he arrives at what I call "the male transcendental orgasm" or MTO. This volcanic explosion is the man's natural, spiritual, sexual moment of enlightenment.

This "thunderbolt climax" may appear to last only thirty seconds to two minutes in chronological time, the average duration being about a minute. What makes this orgasm transcendental is not its external signs, which probably resemble the familiar, and often trivial, male ejaculation. If total surrender on an internal, emotional level is achieved during the climax, if risk-taking to the point of undeniable vulnerability occurs, then a degree of dissolution of the ego mechanism takes place.

The red tantra orgasm path for men evolves into a deeper and deeper letting go into the most central, heartfelt sense of pure identity, of self-in-self, of unbounded awareness or consciousness. More concretely, when his enraptured body is shaking and melting and disappearing under the seductive assault of prolonged sexual arousal, then seems to shoot like a rocket into the clear white light blazing in the heart of a star exploding in a supernova, he may then wonder just exactly who and what and where he really is. Now that's red tantra!

The rough, raw, radical ride on the male orgasmic thunderbolt really does work. It can definitely feel like a life-changing encounter with death. It can and will deliver a rush far greater than he will get parachuting out of a plane.

Many years ago, a Tibetan yogi told me "When I make love to a woman, my prayer is 'May I die in your arms. May my sense of separate self be dissolved in the clear blue bliss-sky of your cosmic wisdom womb. May I die and never return, through the Grace of the Great Mother of All Buddhas.'"

To his wonderful red tantra prayer, all I can add is, "Amen!"

THE RED TANTRA COUPLE

Red tantra works with the sex act exactly as it is. Couples need not change anything. Of course, they can if they wish, but the real import is that they will discover how to see in the forms of fucking, sucking, licking, and masturbating the transcendental formlessness of the Absolute, of Consciousness or God.

If there is not going to be any change on the outside, lovers are left with only one area to create change, and that is the inside. On the outside, then, it will probably look the same. If a friend videotapes you having sex and shows it to an uninitiated couple, to people who have no comprehension of the subtleties of red tantra, she will probably say something like, "Wow! Look at them go. He's really nailing her to the wall!" To which he will add, "Yeah! And she's loving every second of it!"

This doesn't mean, of course, that red tantra has to be hot, hard, and fast. Feel free to unite and then lie quietly in each other's arms, meditating. The point of red tantra is that lovers can do whatever they want!

The key is not on the outside. It is not in the physical movements. It is within. It must be discovered, like learning how to walk or ride a bike.

The inner secret of red tantra is total surrender. She surrenders to her own pleasure, to the red passion flowing hotly through her red blood, to her formless, universal bliss body. I say, "her formless, universal bliss body" because once she has melted into bliss, she will begin to feel formless. If she does not give into the fear of losing her identity, this feeling of ecstatic, vibratory formlessness will open into a deep, spiritual experience of being boundless and universal, in other words, of actually being the Great Goddess whose body is the universe.

He surrenders to her, to her pleasure, and to his own inner death challenge. It is as if he is eager, willing, and able to die on this sacred site for her, to die nobly for a truth and a love deeper and higher and greater than himself.

He is sacrificing his body and psyche on the altar of transcendental truth, which she embodies as the softness and roundness and fullness of love. She is Aphrodite, the essence of beauty's power to attract and inspire.

Then he may experience his sudden, brief, super-intense thunderbolt MTO, just as she experienced her gradual, extended, wave-like, oceanic nirvana orgasm.

THE SECRET POWER OF SELF-PLEASURING

The solo tantrika, male or female, can experience all of this via self-pleasuring. Remember, the pleasure experienced with another, though stimulated by their presence, is not caused by them. This distinction is subtle but crucial.

Perhaps they awakened or aroused or activated the pleasure within, but it had to be inside, innate, on tap in the first place. Otherwise, no amount of stimulation, sexiness, chemistry or anything else from a partner could bring on the experience. A lover can invoke the gift of sexual pleasure. They are powerless to create it.

So, when self-pleasuring, remember this: The source of pleasure is within. The other person may help build the connection to inner power, but they can never be its cause or source. What is the cause of pleasure arising from within? The deeper self. *The Vijnana Bhairava,* a major text of the tantric Kashmir Shaivite school of northern India, advises that "When feelings of pleasure arise, enjoy them in spaciousness, contemplate them with enthusiasm, and trace them back with relentless curiosity to the infinite, luminous, silent source within."

During a solo period several years ago, I remember thinking: "If only I had a partner. My pleasure would be so much greater!" Yet once I got over the psychological obstacle in this assumption, I found that my solo sexual experiences were every bit as rich. My new receptivity made the difference, for nothing else had changed. There were social and sensual interactions that I missed, but the raw sexospiritual glory was not diminished. As I have faced my fears around aloneness and being without a partner or lover, I have discovered an erotic self-sufficiency, a lasting self-love, a source of joy, confidence, and power in my life. Now a sweet completeness permeates everything I do.

As pleasant as it can be to have a partner for tantric play, the reality is that often the other person becomes an energy drain. They may have boosted the tantrika's energy in the beginning, during the romance stage, but now they are taking it from them. Of course, not all relationships are like this. Some actually work!

Whether a tantrika is in a relationship or not, the relationship with self is the primary one. It must always be honored. Lovers come and go. Even marriage is no longer a guarantee. It is in your best interest to take total responsibility for your sexual pleasure, your tantric journey and, ultimately, your self-realization.

Nonetheless, it is natural to want to be in a relationship. Some people come to me for counseling because they want to find a partner. I tell them "Pleasure yourself several times a week. Have a blast doing it. Enjoy the pleasure more than ever before. Try new things and be inventive. Sooner or later, somebody will notice you!"

Of course, what often happens is they start having so much fun with themselves, they forget all about looking for somebody. Then they're shopping for groceries or doing the laundry or taking a yoga class and—boom!—there is the person they were looking for standing in front of them.

HOW TO GET MORE FROM THIS BOOK

It was a beautiful spring afternoon in the Pacific Northwest. I was in a Borders bookstore and happened upon a book by the respected sex therapist Lonnie Barbach. It combined the erotic stories of another author with her own abundant sexual insights. In a flash, I knew how to approach *Red Hot Tantra*.

My co-author would write stories that conveyed the rich, complex, elusive feelings, textures, vibrations, sounds, and colors of tantra. I would then follow these stories with guided spiritual experiences and insightful, friendly commentaries. These red tantra instructions and insights would leave no doubt that a radical spiritual awakening is possible via conscious, loving sexual encounters like those described in the erotic stories.

There are twenty-two erotic, red "Tantric Tales" by Cynthia W. Gentry in *Red Hot Tantra*. Each is accompanied by a "Tantric Experience." I would like you to think that each tantric erotic story needs the tantric experience or commentary that goes with it to complete it. The stories are the yin and the experiences are the yang, and it is only in their complete fusion that the greater meaning of each is revealed. The stories speak to the artistic, intuitive right brain while the guided experiences and commentaries address the logical, linear left brain.

As you read *Red Hot Tantra*, you will learn that tantra is like a holy fire. Fire gives off heat, movement, and light. The erotic stories are the heat. The experiences are the movement of the flames. Together, they produce light.

I suggest that you first read a story, then set the book aside to absorb its impact. See if you can arrive at your own red-tantric insights by deeply feeling and inwardly attuning with it. Then read the experience section. If you resonate with the experience, if you find yourself feeling excited about exploring this technique, I encourage you to do it as soon as possible. The positive feeling response is a sign that it holds a gift for you.

Tantra teaches that human beings are always seeking the highest possible pleasure because the pure essence of pleasure reflects their true nature. In Sanskrit, this pure pleasure at the source of being, experienced vividly in the peak of the sexual orgasm, is known as "ananda," or unconditional bliss.

For more information about goddess worship, cervical orgasm, and other topics vital to the practice of red tantra, please see the Red Hot Resources guide at the end of this book. There I have listed and described the books, tapes, tools, toys, and Web sites that my research has shown to be the best available.

CHAPTER TWO

2

Tantric Meditation

TANTRIC TALE

Surrender

WHEN PAUL FINALLY LOOKS UP FROM THE BOOK, I'm not sure whether I want to laugh in his face or slap it. It's his expression that gets to me: that patient, gentle expression I've seen most often on our gray cat, Chuck, who now lies dozing by the fireplace. Paul looks at me for another moment, as though he knows what I'm thinking and doesn't care, and then goes back to the book. *It's a book on Tantric sex,* I want to scream. *Not a gardening manual. Can't you show a little more interest?*

"You don't have to read the whole thing," I say. I try, somewhat unsuccessfully, to keep the impatience out of my voice. "Just the parts I highlighted."

He flips to a part of the book that I know I didn't mark.

"Not that part, sweetie. The part I highlighted."

"I know what you highlighted." He continues reading.

I let out my breath in a short, quick exhale that he ought to know by now is my signal of extreme exasperation.

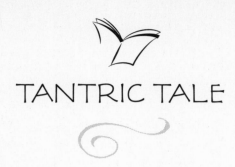

"That's good," he says without looking up. With his head bent over the book, his black, shoulder-length hair obscures his face. I can tell by his tone that he's smiling. "The book says that breathing is good."

I get up from the couch, stalk to the bedroom, and flop onto the bed. The rich texture of the blue velvet duvet cover—a color and texture I chose for its soothing properties—fails to comfort me. What was I thinking, bringing home a book on Tantric sex? Sure, when I'd glanced through it at the bookstore, I'd had high hopes that it would hold the secret to putting some spice back into our sex life, a sex life that has grown predictable and missionary over the eight years of our marriage. But it was Paul's dependability and gentleness that had attracted me to him in the first place. He was the antidote to my type A personality, his quiet stubbornness the complement to my mercurial moods. He had calmed my neuroses, softened my rough edges. And he had been the first man to be able to make me climax. Falling in love with him had been like easing myself into a warm bath. But as the years went by and I found myself organizing our lives more and more—from planning our weekly dinner menus to organizing vacations—resentment had seeped into my heart like an underground spring of ice cold water, freezing my libido. Paul hadn't been able to make me come for months.

Now, I bury my face into the duvet cover and try to think of what to do next. *He's not going to get it,* I think. *It's not going to work*. I feel tears well up in my eyes. I'm so tired, I think. Tired of doing everything.

Suddenly I feel his hand on the small of my back. I'm about to flip over and bat it away when he speaks.

"Hold still."

Then, before I can move, he's tied a blindfold over my eyes. *Where the hell did he get that?* I wonder.

"Turn over. Lie still."

He pulls my tank top over my head, and slides my yoga pants over my hips and down my legs. I'm seized with the urge to giggle, to crack a joke, to put myself back on top. But just as I start to open my mouth, he stops touching me. The absence of his hand is like a shock, a blast of cold air.

"Where'd you go?" I ask.

"Be quiet."

I hear the scratch of a match, and through the blindfold, I can sense that he's lit candles. I smell cinnamon and sandalwood. Then I feel the bed sink under his weight as he stretches out beside me.

"I want you to breathe, Mary. Breathe through your entire body. From the top of your head to your toes. Every pore."

If I want to do breathing exercises, I'll go to yoga class, I almost say, but then I find myself taking long, slow, deep breaths anyway. He begins to coach me, his lips close to my ear.

"Relax," he whispers. "That's a good girl."

I feel a stirring between my legs, an electric twinge inside. It takes me by surprise.

"Keep breathing like that. No matter what I do."

I'm starting to feel a little lightheaded, but I keep breathing.

Then he begins touching me. I feel as though a stranger's hands are caressing my body. He starts stroking me lightly, up and down my legs. His fingers dance around my parted thighs. I start to reach for his hand to put his fingers on my sex. *Let's get this party started,* I think. But he pushes my hand away.

"You may not move your hands," he says, as stern as any headmaster. I obey.

He begins stroking my stomach. I want to double over and protect myself, but I can't. I try to breathe. Then he encircles my breasts, brushing his fingers over my nipples.

This isn't in the book, I want to say. *This wasn't what I highlighted.*

"Keep breathing," he says, as if reading my mind. His fingers brush over my neck, my face, my eyelids, my lips. Then he returns to my nipples. He frets them gently at first, increasing the pressure slowly. He replaces his fingers with his tongue, which flicks back and forth over one nipple, then the other. I imagine that tongue between my legs. But it's his fingers that travel over my stomach and, finally, find their home between my thighs.

I tense. What if, after all this, I still can't come?

But his fingers refuse to entertain that as a possibility. They reach my clit and press hard, insistently. "Relax," he whispers again in my ear. "Let it come to you."

I begin, involuntarily, to rock my hips, thrusting to meet his fingers.

"Don't move. Don't. Move." His voice sounds almost angry. "Don't *do* anything. Just feel. Just breathe. If you start to think about something else, let the thought float away. Just breathe."

"But . . ."

"Let it come to you."

I feel my body go limp and yet become aroused at the same time. His finger is moving over my clit faster and faster. I can tell how wet I am by the slippery sound his finger makes. He shifts his weight and suddenly, he's on top of me. I feel his hardness touch the lips of my soft wetness.

"I want you inside me," I whisper.

"When I'm ready." His finger keeps moving on my clit. I feel him beginning to slide in, a quarter-inch at a time. "Keep breathing," he says.

He is completely inside me now, but somehow he's maneuvering it so that he's still able to rub my clit. My skin is tingling. I'm not exactly sure what's happening.

"I'm going to do anything I want to you," he whispers in my ear. "Will you do exactly what I say?"

"Yes." I'm not sure whether I've answered or not. He's thrusting into me rhythmically, totally in control of his movements, the pace, the depth. I feel him all the way inside me, up to my womb. He allows me to match his thrusts, and I feel as though we're fusing. Some part of me notices that the pace of our breathing matches. It's as though he's injecting me with waves of electricity.

And then something happens that I'm at a loss to explain. I feel my *self*—my angry, frustrated, insistent self—separate out. It is suddenly only on the surface of me. And I realize that all my efforts to control Paul, to change and to manage him, have been efforts to take *his* self over, to envelop him like some amorphous, needy protoplasm. What I needed was to let my deepest self—the part that can trust and surrender and totally let go—take *me* over. I have been trying to change who he is. But I just needed to be who I am, all of who I am, even those depths in my soul that have no name.

I stop thinking, and let myself feel. I am on the verge of climaxing. I want to come. I am so close. I try to stave it off. He seems to sense it, but he doesn't slow or change his pace.

"You can come now," he says.

All I can hear is his voice. I feel as though I'm falling and rising at the same time, and I clutch my legs around him to hang on. My outer self, the part that's always in charge, crackles and burns up and flies away like pieces of vellum turned to ash. My protective shell is gone, but Paul will not hurt me. I hand myself to him, trusting him now, the scar tissue gone to reveal glowing fresh skin.

And still he thrusts against me with the same rhythm, his finger on my clit. He pulls my blindfold away and dares me—forces me—to look into his violet eyes, the pupils as large and black as moons. He takes his other hand and slips it under my butt. His fingers graze the tight opening.

The orgasm starts in my toes as he thrusts harder and harder. Waves of current flash up and down my body. He no longer needs to touch my clit. From someplace far away, my true self hears my earthbound self screaming in pleasure.

When the orgasm subsides and I return to earth, Paul is holding me. There's no need for me to speak. I notice that my face is cool from my evaporated tears. My tears? Where did the tears come from? But Paul lets me cry. I'm mourning, but I'm happy, too, truly content for this brief moment. For the first time in my life, I realize that I am not alone.

TANTRIC EXPERIENCE

Remember the Spaciousness

TANTRA IS, ABOVE ALL ELSE, A PATH OF EXPERIENCE. When you are in the thralls of sexual passion, you probably focus on the pleasurable sensations. Have you ever noticed the space around them? Have you ever noticed that your sexual feelings are taking place inside of an openness? This may sound abstract. Or you may think that noticing the space around your pleasure will not add to it.

In fact, becoming aware of the space gives the pleasure room to expand. In other words, you will be able to feel more deeply, and what you will feel will be even more beautiful than before.

Please let me take you on a journey so that you can experience this. Sit or lie down in a comfortable position. It is best if the telephone is turned off. Peaceful music is a possibility if you prefer some kind of sound.

Please return to a moment of intensely beautiful sexual pleasure. It can be an experience of orgasm, but it doesn't have to be.

Perhaps you were alone. Perhaps you were with a partner.

Please go back there now.

See what there is to see. Listen to the sounds. Smell the fragrances. Be in the textures of touching. Feel the feelings in your body. Notice how you are breathing. Do you feel good thinking about this memory? Ideally, the feeling you get thinking about this memory will not be mixed or confusing for you in any way. It will be pure, pleasant, and uplifting, like the fragrance of a rose.

Check with your body. Notice the pure, good, pleasurable feeling in your body now. This is a memory, so the feeling is subtle.

Relive the joys that you explored in your tantra, in the orgasm, in the loving, sensuous surrenders to light and hair and perfume and sound, in the wetness and dreaminess and closeness and helplessness. Breathe, remember, celebrate the sweet erotic feelings, the warm, wide open, flowing, glowing, expanded feelings, in your body now. Notice that there is a rich feeling of openness associated with this pleasure that is now spreading through your whole body.

Now gently, tenderly focus on that relaxed, open spaciousness. Allow it to expand like a colorful party balloon. Allow the openness of the pleasure to expand completely.

It is expanding the way a flower opens all its petals—slowly, in a natural way, and completely.

Notice the pleasure.
Notice the space.
Notice the luminosity of this pleasurable space.
Notice the silence of this pleasurable space.
Notice the depth of this pleasurable space.
Let go of all thoughts.
Allow yourself to float, to flow, to flower.
Allow yourself to be.
Just be.
When you are ready, return to this now.
At your own pace, return to this time and place here.
Welcome back.
Did you enjoy that?

Tantra teaches vivid wakefulness in expanded states of pleasure.

All of your positive, pleasurable sexual experiences can be subjects for meditation. Where there is pleasure, there is spaciousness. In this spaciousness, there is less ego, less fear, less contraction.

Through meditation, you can become more awake, alert and aware inside of this spaciousness. This will lead you to freedom.

Yet pleasure tends to lull you to sleep, to forgetfulness, to vagueness. This is the ordinary relationship to pleasure: To use it like a drug, like a sleeping pill, to have it comfort you and put you back to sleep. Consciousness does not wake up in people just because they have sex. You and I know that!

How do you stay awake and aware in the midst of intense pleasure? Perhaps the closest that words can come is this: Let go totally, surrender completely, then just be. Leave nothing behind, not even yourself.

I suggest that you begin your tantric journey with surrender. Surrender with respect and reverence to your partner, to your deep self, to life, to death, to love, to truth, to God, to the universe, to that which is greater than you.

In the beginning of this journey, you discover that you can be more open. Eventually, you realize that you are the openness. These insights blossom into a source of great joy. Sexual freedom is sex as an experience of freedom. This is the tantric view.

Tantra says these moments are valuable. These are teachings about who you are when you are in an optimal, expanded state. Sexual arousal, orgasm, afterglow—these are all high, altered states with power to create insight, healing, transformation, bliss. They are life's gifts. Use them.

You can recall these special moments as an ever-present resource. As you relax your need to control, you realize your demand for control is based on fear. You discover that you can "go to zero," as one meditation teacher put it. You can't do it every time, but you can go to zero, relax into the openness, when you really need to do it.

You push less and absorb more. You are more skillful in difficult situations. You respond to essentials instead of reacting to fantasies.

You discover how to let go. Specifically, you discover how to let go in the here and now, when you are in the thick of it, while you are caught up in the action of life. By leaving no residue, no remnant, you find the center at the heart of the action. This center in the midst of action is like the eye of a hurricane: silent, mysterious, motionless, magnificent.

As your experience of letting go and finding the restful center in the midst of action deepens, your capacity to enjoy life deepens as well. Gratitude and appreciation permeate your mind. Your tantric surrender turns into a treasure that enriches your whole life. This discovery of the solid, nourishing ground of openness, and of your growing identity with it, is the beginning.

With ego-death, there is also surrender. Only there is not the coming back. The universe takes you in its arms and never lets go. You melt back into its infinite body, which is your source. You return to where you began. It is the final orgasm of the ego, the ultimate surrender, after which no more surrender is possible or needed. Or it could be said that surrender is now so natural, that it is like breathing. Either way, when it happens, it just simply happens.

In the story, Paul and Mary enter the great way. Paul surrenders and finds his power. Mary surrenders and discovers her vulnerability. Hard and soft, power and vulnerability, form and emptiness—in the dance of the Tao, they find each other.

TANTRIC TALE

Loving-Kindness

CHARLES' WIFE SUSAN HAS BEGUN DROPPING THINGS: plates, food, her keys. When he's feeling more compassionate, Charles chuckles and reminds her about staying focused and in the moment. Other times, despite his best intentions, he snaps at her to pay attention. Whether he's losing patience or she's becoming clumsier, he's not sure. At any rate, he isn't totally surprised when, late one night, he hears the sound of breaking china from the kitchen. He finds her with her back to the sink, breathing hard. Her hands, clad in yellow rubber gloves, hang at her sides as though they, too, are waiting for his reaction.

"What did you drop this time?" he asks. He thinks about the unfinished e-mail on his computer, the cursor blinking at him, waiting for him as well.

Susan stares at him with a look that occupies the no-man's land between panic and rage, a look that always frightens him deeply. His heart sinks. *Here we go,* he thinks.

"I told you I just had a few more e-mails to write," he says.

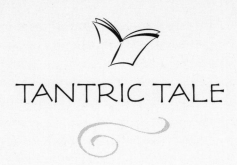

That's when he sees the brown liquid dripping from the wall opposite the sink. He recognizes this liquid as his after-dinner tea. His eyes follow its trail to the floor, where an explosion of white porcelain lies on the carpet. His face goes cold and begins to tingle. He has never before seen anything approaching violence from her.

"It slipped," she says in a tiny voice. "I'm sorry. I'm sorry."

"Bullshit. It didn't slip." He's afraid to approach her. She reminds him of the cornered horse he saw on a public television show about branding. As the horse's owner had approached with the red-hot iron, the horse had lashed out with its hooves, nearly missing the owner's head.

"I have to tell you something," Susan says. "You need to pay attention."

He starts to say, *There are better ways to get my attention,* when he realizes that she is continuing to talk. And then he realizes what she is telling him. With each word, she changes his life, her words like hooves kicking his face, his chest, his heart. He reaches out to keep himself from falling, but there is nothing there. Suddenly, she is beside him, leading him to a chair in the dining room.

She tells him that she needs him out of the house for a few days and hands him a paper with the addresses of a few meditation centers. "At least one of them must be having a retreat this weekend," she tells him, not unkindly. "Time for you to practice what you preach."

When the thought crosses his mind that she is getting him out of the house so that she can see her lover, she says, pre-empting his comments, "I told you. It happened once and then it was over. I was a conquest. All I want now is to be alone for a little bit. Okay?"

And that's how, a few days later, Charles finds himself sitting on a small round cushion in a room with twenty other people. He can hardly remember how he got here; he vaguely remembers packing a few things into his gym bag while Susan was at her shrink's, getting into his car, and starting it. The next thing he knew, he was on a winding highway high above the ocean. He remembers trying to keep his car along the center line, because he was afraid that if he allowed himself to look out at the water, he would point the car towards it, and he is quite certain that if he had dashed his car on the rocks below, he would have come back in his next life as a sea slug.

But even now, as he sits in this room on a cliff overlooking the magnificent California coastline, his mind wanders outside. He quickly reminds himself that he is Not Suicidal. He brings himself back to The Moment. Good.

A tall, thin, dark-haired man enters the room and sits at the front of the class. He emanates such warmth that Charles wants to cry. Charles could imagine having a beer with this man, and in fact, wishes he were.

"We're going to do the loving-kindness meditation today," the teacher says. "This is also known as the Buddhist meditation 'metta.' It really is very simple. We are going to be sending loving-kindness energy, full of unconditional love, out to ourselves, our loved ones, and the world."

Oh, bullshit, Charles thinks. *Just what I need. To send kind thoughts to the wife who cheated on me and hates me. Like that's gonna work.* He sees Susan at the sink with those rubber gloves, preparing to slice him open with her words. But then other images flash through his mind like a rapid-fire slideshow: Susan fixing him gourmet meals from recipes in magazines. Buying him little gifts, like a gift certificate from his favorite record store. Sending him text messages on his cell phone that read like a child's hieroglyphics: *Luv u. Miss u. Want 2 kiss u.* Her naked body under him, how it felt to be inside her, exploring her wetness, her mouth on him.

The slideshow continues with images that make Charles cringe with regret: him telling Susan that her orgasms were her responsibility. That it didn't matter if they were making love less frequently because their relationship was about more than just sex. He sees himself at his computer, long after she has stopped waiting up for him. He has an image of himself climbing into bed beside her at two in the morning and reaching for her warm body, of her reaching for his flaccid penis, of her spooning into him and falling asleep.

"Open your child's mind, your innocent mind, and be surprised and delighted," the teacher is saying. "And for the next five minutes, simply repeat to yourself, 'May I be happy.'"

Charles bursts into tears.

When he comes back from the retreat, he and Susan are like strangers who have suddenly found themselves to be roommates. Susan, who carries herself with a sort of resigned guilt, seems to expect nothing from him. They sleep in the same bed, but without touching. They treat each other with aching politeness. Charles is sure that by the end of the month, Susan will ask him to move out for good. But that weekend, they are invited to a party at the home of some friends, and to his surprise, Susan says she wants to go. He wonders how he will be able to act normally.

As Charles is dressing, he catches sight of Susan in the bathroom as she applies her makeup. She wears a simple black lace thong and a black bra. Typical Susan: nothing frilly, nothing lacy. She doesn't need lace to take attention away from the curve of her hip, the roundness of her thighs, the swelling of her small breasts. He watches her brush her long black hair as she gazes into the mirror. He knows she is not even looking at her own reflection. Her thoughts are somewhere else. At one point, he used to have an idea of what she was thinking.

At the party, he watches her as though he's never seen her before. The words of the meditation teacher flit across his brain: *Open your child's mind, and let yourself be surprised and delighted.* Charles watches Susan move across the room, her hips swaying. She should have been a runway model, he thinks. Then she goes to pour herself a glass of wine and the liquid sloshes out onto the white lace tablecloth. She looks up quickly to see whether she's been observed. Charles catches her eye, and they grin at each other. Co-conspirators. She moves a plate to cover the stain, and Charles has to cover his mouth to keep from laughing.

She walks over to him.

"What will you give me not to tell?" he whispers to her.

"What do you want?" she asks, and inside his pants, he feels himself stiffen. He leans in to kiss her, and she presses herself against him.

"Get a room, you two," a guy walking by says, laughing. They ignore him.

When they get home, they make it as far as the living room. Charles lowers Susan to the couch as if she were made of porcelain. He removes her shoes, then her dress. He unsnaps her bra, sets it aside, and takes a moment to cup her breasts in his hands. He kisses them one at a time. He can't believe how beautiful they are, how round, how soft, how perfect. How had he forgotten this?

"I'm sorry," he whispers. "I'm so sorry." His eyes fill with tears that overflow the corners of his eyes. She wipes them away.

"I am too," she says. "But I'm back. Forever."

He kisses her rib cage, her belly button, and then the soft curve of her stomach. He slips his fingers under her panties and pulls them down over her legs. He runs a gentle finger over the smooth folds of her womanhood. It swells under his touch. He covers it with his mouth and begins to lick her from her opening to her clitoris and back again. Moaning, she arches her back, and after a few minutes, she reaches for him. But he won't let her stop him.

"It's OK," he whispers. "Just relax. Let me pay attention to you."

He presses her hands down beside her and continues to lick her, teasing her with the tip of his tongue. He drapes her legs over his shoulders and loses himself in her. He redoubles his efforts, his tongue relentless. He hears her breathing quicken and feels her muscles stiffen. Suddenly, she comes, arching against him and crying out.

"I have to have you inside me," she moans. "Please, honey."

He quickly removes his clothes and pulls her up onto him. He can't believe how good it feels inside her. He holds her hips to his, never taking his eyes off her flushed face.

"Do you know how much I love you?" he asks.

She shakes her head.

"This much," he says, taking his hands off her momentarily to spread them as far as they will go. She smiles, her face shining, and he realizes how much he has missed the light in her eyes. *May you be happy,* he thinks. *May we be happy.*

As she rocks against him, he feels the orgasm build and then burst inside him. He comes harder than he has in months, but he keeps his eyes open. He doesn't want to miss a thing about her, ever again.

TANTRIC EXPERIENCE

Loving-Kindness Meditation

LOVING-KINDNESS IS A CLASSIC BUDDHIST MEDITATION. It has been around for a long time—more than 2,500 years. Surprisingly, you hear little about it outside of Buddhist circles.

Like any great meditation technique, loving-kindness can be approached simply with good results. Traditionally, this meditation is called *metta*. So, if you said to a traditional Buddhist, "I would like to do metta for my friend who is in the hospital," he or she would know exactly what you mean: You are going to radiate loving-kindness energy to that person in need.

Obviously, you can't do loving-kindness meditation—let's just call it "metta," it's shorter—for others if you can't do it for yourself. You can't share what you don't have.

The beauty of metta is that you can start right where you are. If you keep it up, you will experience more and more pure, true, real love in your life.

In fact, the Buddha listed no less than eleven benefits from doing metta. Metta puts a glow on your features, so that you are beautiful regardless of your physical characteristics. Metta makes you popular, too. You gain charisma, plenty of good friends, and a charming personality. In fact, because you're putting out such good vibes, the Buddha said metta would even improve your luck and good fortune in life. Plus it helps you go to sleep and to sleep deeply when you do.

When you do metta meditation, you want to be as comfortable as possible. I don't care about the outer attitude of your body. I do care about the inner attitude of your mind and heart.

First, take a few minutes just to breathe in a relaxed way. Nothing fancy. Just breathe in a little more deeply than you usually do. When you breathe out, let it feel like a sweet sigh. Allow a gentle half-smile. Have you ever wondered what the essence of love is? According to the Buddha, it is the wish or intent "May you be happy!" When you do metta, you always start with yourself. In fact, some days that's all you will do. You will just love yourself nonstop for twenty minutes!

So, get comfortable. Repeat to yourself with sincere feeling, "May I be happy. May I be happy. May I be happy."

Use a soft, warm, gentle tone of voice. Television's Mr. Rogers of "Welcome to my neighborhood!" fame had a voice infused with metta. That he was popular and beloved around the world was no accident.

Focus on the center of your chest area. That is where your spiritual heart is. Focus right there, in the middle of your chest, and encourage that area to soften, open and unfold, like a golden flower. Relax and melt into any good feelings that may arise.

Remember the song "Happy Together" by the Turtles? It is still popular decades later. That's what everybody wants in a relationship. What better foundation can there be than a heartfelt wish for happiness for each other?

After you and your partner do a few solo metta sessions, it's time to do metta together. Smile! Say the words, "May I be happy!" silently. Doing "May I be happy!" is the first step.

Now that your special friend is here doing metta with you, you would like them to be happy, too. From their point of view, this also means they have exactly the same wish for you. The second step of metta is "May you be happy!"

After you've warmed up the love energy in your own heart, take turns sending the loving-kindness energy to each other. One of you volunteers to start sharing metta. They say "May you be happy!" out loud with a soft, warm, gentle tone of voice. After a few minutes, switch roles. The sender is now the receiver. In a relaxed, easy-going way, the new sender now intentionally radiates metta.

Now you're both in the beautiful metta space. The third and final step is to share this love vibration with the world, or at least let it expand out from your love zone.

Does this sound enjoyable? I hope so. For years I led groups of up to fifteen people doing exactly this. Metta is, as the joke goes, the most fun you can have with your clothes on!

The third and final step is "May everybody be happy!" Take the warm glow that you've created together and share it with the world. If a friend or family member needs support, then focus on them. Out loud, together, say three times (or more), "May everybody be happy!" Here, the whole world is meant. This is akin to praying for world peace. After you get comfortable with the "be happy" phrases, replace them with this short, powerful sentence that covers most life issues: "May I/You/Everybody be happy, healthy, peaceful, prosperous, and free!"

Do you want to send metta to your Aunt Amelia who is in the hospital? It's easy. "May Aunt Amelia be happy, healthy, peaceful, prosperous, and free!"

Loving-kindness is like a muscle—the more you use it, the stronger it gets.

Do just twenty minutes of metta twice a week. You will be impressed, maybe amazed, by the results. If love is the answer, then metta is a timeless, proven way to change lives and improve intimate relationships with the heart.

In the story, Charles and Susan discover that the invisible glue holding them together is greater than they are. In their crisis, they uncover a magnificent mystery that words like love, kindness, caring, respect, gratitude, compassion describe but do not contain—the depths of the human heart.

Let's take a moment to thank the Buddha for this great meditation.

"Lord Buddha, may you be happy, healthy, peaceful, prosperous, and free!"

TANTRIC TALE

No Ego

THE TAPE ARRIVES IN A SMALL WHITE CARDBOARD BOX ON the last Wednesday of the month. Jennifer stands at the mailbox, holding the small package as if it were a bird's nest. For a moment, she does not feel the September sun on her skin, nor see the maple leaves that are just beginning to turn crimson and gold. She does not hear the laughter of her neighbor's four-year-old across the street as he plays hide-and-seek with his older sister. She does not hear the cars on South Bedford Road, nor realize that it is late afternoon in upstate New York. She simply stares at the box and its return address, and imagines that she is on another coast, in a place on a cliff far above the ocean, a place where the Monterey pines are so bent by the wind that their branches look like the arms of old men in prayer.

Then she shakes her head. *Daydreaming again,* she says to herself. *Can't you live life in the present, even for an instant?*

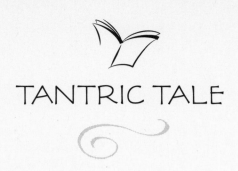

She walks up the gravel path to her cottage. Once inside, she draws the curtain in the living room: first the ivory silk panels, then the heavy burgundy drapes. The room becomes as dark as night, as dark as a womb. Jennifer sits on a square cushion in the corner of the room and opens the box. The tape lies inside it like a pearl, swaddled in bubble wrap. She puts it in the tape deck, hits play, and shuts her eyes.

CDs would sound so much better, the voice in her head says. *Stop it, monkey mind,* she tells the voice. *I'm meditating.*

Then the tape starts, and a new voice fills the room. Sharon's voice.

Welcome. Greetings to you who cannot be with us in person. Greetings to the deep self.

Jennifer breathes deeply, in and out. She leaves behind the clinic. The crying children. The pain. She puts them on a lily pad in the river of her thoughts, gives them a push, and watches them drift downstream. She returns to Sharon's voice.

Since you are an advanced student of meditation, this month I would like to discuss an advanced subject. Sexual climax meditation. Since we at the Blue Sky Meditation School do not practice celibacy, I am assuming that most of you have orgasms.

Jennifer opens her eyes. She feels herself tense in surprise. She has never heard Sharon discuss sex before, and she's not sure she's comfortable with it.

First, I want to clarify a misconception about the mechanics of achieving the orgasm. Intercourse between two people is often assumed to be the most intimate, ideal way to achieve sexual orgasm for spiritual purposes.

Based on my own experience and feedback from students, I've found that this is not true. If your goal is to work with the sexual orgasm as a state of meditation, an orgasm achieved via masturbation with a vibrator or the hand or other methods works just as well. In fact, these methods may minimize ego static by reducing self-consciousness. The ideal orgasm meditation may be a scenario where the meditator is pleasured to climax without any expectation of immediate reciprocation.

Jennifer's heart begins to pound. She strains to understand Sharon's words.

When you explore the orgasm as a state of meditation, you are not seeking to bond or merge with another human being. If it happens, allow it. Then return to your focus on yourself. Merging with another person may or may not bring you any closer to your deep, true self. In fact, merging with another person may take you further away from it.

Jennifer forces her mind to think calm thoughts, then wonders whether something is wrong if she has to force her mind to do anything. She remembers a late-night garden conversation at Blue Sky where she tried to talk to Sharon, in her roundabout way, about her sexual problems. Sharon had told her, simply but with compassion, to be patient with herself. "More will be revealed," she said with a smile. And Jennifer has tried, through a move to the East Coast, a new job, and several disastrous dates, to be patient. But now she is confused. Isn't the whole point of sex to bond with another person? *I want to know why I can't bond,* Jennifer says to the Sharon on the tape.

Now we are going to explore this state of meditation. Please feel free to stop the tape now or at any time if you wish. Respect where you are now.

Jennifer reaches over to the tape deck, but her hand stops in mid-air. She returns it to her lap. She is not sure whether she is curious or frightened, but she has always trusted her meditation teacher.

Do whatever you need to do to make yourself comfortable.

Jennifer pauses the tape. She hesitates, and then strips off her drawstring pants. She reminds herself that no one can see her; the door is locked. She feels silly sitting there bottomless, so she pulls her T-shirt over her head. What the heck, she tries to tell herself. *Listening to a tape can't hurt me.*

She takes some pillows from the couch and arranges them around her. She lights a candle on the mantelpiece and stares, for a moment, at her face in the mirror above the fireplace. She pulls the ponytail holder out of her hair and watches her dark blonde hair frame her face. *I look tired,* she thinks. She tries to avoid looking at her body. Instead she sits back down on the cushions, and leans back into them.

Touch yourself, starting at the top of your head. Feel the softness of your hair. Caress your earlobes. Stroke the curves of your cheekbones. Run your fingertips over your features as if you were a blind man memorizing the features of a loved one.

Touch your neck and feel your pulse beating. Know that you are alive. Feel every curve, every protuberance. Touch your breasts.

Jennifer hesitates. But then she moves the palms of her hands over her nipples. She begins to move her hands in circles around her nipples until they are hard. She nearly misses the next part of the tape.

Move your hands lower. Caress the ribs that protect your heart. Feel your waist. Carefully touch your belly. Your hipbones. Breathe. Discover your skin.

She does.

Touch the tops of your thighs.

Now, when you're ready, touch yourself between your legs. Play with your pubic hair, if you want. Feel its coarseness. When you're ready, touch your clitoris. Rediscover the folds around it.

Jennifer's throat hurts. This is how a lover should be touching me, she thinks, if I didn't scare them all away, even the one that wanted to marry me. *All the time and money spent on fucking meditation retreats, and I'm still alone with myself.*

She forces herself to look at the thought, then let go of it. It floats away from her like a bubble on a stream, and then evaporates. She watches it, surprised. She didn't think it would be so easy.

She realizes that she is still moving her fingers over her clitoris. She is confused, but she does not stop. *What, do I have to masturbate every time I meditate? Or vice versa?* She watches that thought, too, drift away.

But then she notices that she is becoming aroused, wet. She dips a finger down, into her vagina, to make sure. Yes, she is swollen, wide, soft. She knows that she is on the path to orgasm, and she is afraid of the thoughts that will follow.

But it's too late.

She sees herself being pushed onto a bed, face down. She smells beer. She hears her father's voice, laughing roughly.

She shakes violently. She pulls her hands away from her body and slams them to the floor. No, she will not masturbate, even though she is so aroused now that it hurts. She will not orgasm, and she will not have to run to the bathroom afterwards, her stomach heaving. No orgasm, no vomit. No orgasm, no broken engagement. No orgasm, no dumped fiancé.

Why was Sharon doing this to her? Jennifer wonders whether the fact that a woman's voice has aroused her means she is gay. But then she hears Sharon's words.

Notice the thoughts that arise. Let them go. If you need to, stop the tape and follow your breathing, in and out. When you're ready, touch yourself again. Keep yourself in the sensations.

Jennifer obeys. She notices her thoughts, puts them on the lily pad, and gives them a push. She watches them float away. She breathes for what seems like hours. She begins rubbing herself again, faster. One hands steals up to her nipple, and her fingers begin making quick circles around it until it becomes hard. She begins to feel the pulsing that signals her orgasm.

Pay close attention to the peak. The exact instant of the least ego—of no ego— is the moment of the most bliss. The intensity of the orgasm temporarily overcomes the surface self like a giant wave inundating a tiny sand castle left by a child on the beach. This allows the deep self to emerge, the deep self whose nature is real bliss, real love, real freedom. Orgasm is a direct, undiluted taste of the deep self. The beauty of sexual orgasm is that it shows you just how joyful it is to live without resistance, to let go of fear and surrender to total, unbounded aliveness.

You put your energy into pushing instead of relaxing and receiving. How can life be anything but a struggle if you believe that your everyday life is a fight?

Jennifer eases the pressure on her clitoris for a moment to keep herself from coming. She is not sure that she wants her deeper self to emerge, but it is too late now.

Outside, your orgasm will look the same. Inside, it will be a spiritual initiation. Do not try to kill the ego. You cannot win a battle against something that doesn't exist. Instead, discover and drink deeply of the higher joy of letting go. Study the mystery of surrender. Build the courage to face your fears, your shame, your self-hatred. Let go. Let go. Let go. Then let go some more. The more deeply you surrender, the higher your pleasure. Deeper surrender, higher pleasure.

Jennifer repeats these words as she rubs herself harder and harder. She takes the finger from her nipple and slides it into her wet vagina. She can't hold back any longer. She lets go. Her legs stiffen and her toes point. Suddenly it is as if she sees the sun. As the orgasm takes over, she feels as though she is exploding, her back arching to the sky. For a moment she is suspended, and she feels the orgasm's energy radiate out from her body. She is aware of everything around her at the same moment she feels herself disappear. Sharon's soothing voice continues to speak.

Your deep self, your true self, is always here. At the moment of orgasm, the clouds part to reveal the sun. The sun is always shining. Contemplate these words during meditation and when you enter the orgasmic state.

Jennifer can barely hear the words. She feels as though her body has become the sun. The orgasm keeps rippling through her body longer than she thought possible, filling her with warmth. Finally, it subsides. She is filled with a sense of safety, as though she were cradled in her mother's arms.

On the tape, a quiet gong sounds once, then twice. It marks the end of the meditation. Jennifer lets the tape play to the end. She wiggles her fingers and toes, and stretches her arms above her head. She knows exactly where she is. With a serenity she didn't know she possessed, she rises from her cushion and goes to her bedroom. She slides under her cool white sheets. Her cat jumps onto the bed and curls next to her, and begins to purr.

For the first time in many months, Jennifer falls asleep instantly. Her river of thoughts subsides, eddies, and then flows into a watercourse of graceful dreams, dreams in which wizened pines grow side by side with crimson-blooming maples.

TANTRIC EXPERIENCE

Orgasmic Supernova

THE SEXUAL ORGASM IS A PERSONAL TASTE OF THE BLISS OF space. Your sexual climax is not just a physical event. Your energy field is also deeply involved and affected.

To experience your energy field, imagine a transparent bubble all around your body at a distance of three feet. You can make it out of gold or rainbows or sparkling diamonds. After all, it is your energy field!

With your eyes open, try to sense or feel the edges of your energy field bubble. Then, with your eyes closed, look at the inside of your forehead for any images of your energy field. Finally, with eyes open or closed, listen for the unique vibrations of your personal energy bubble.

Now begin to stimulate yourself using your preferred means. After you have become aroused, check with your bubble. What is happening to it? Is it vibrating faster? Is it flashing colors? Is it making music? Continue the stimulation. Check on your eroticized energy field several times. Many changes are possible, so I won't try to list them here. I can assure you, though, that your energy field is pulsating faster and shining brighter than it was before you started self-pleasuring.

As you approach orgasm, you have several options with this method. You can focus on the edge of your energy field with your feelings. You can close your eyes and look at the forehead for images and visions. You can listen for vibrations, perhaps a kind of angelic music or the hum of bees.

Or you can scan through the body and locate an area, such as the genitals, heart or top of the head, which is doing more than its share of "melting." That is, due to the intense sexual arousal, that area of the body no longer feels dense and solid to you. Instead, it has taken on a kind of liquid or flowing quality. If you find such an area, focus on it during your climax.

The common ingredient in all of these options is concentration. Once you have chosen your focus, keep your attention exclusively on it as you enter your climax, enjoy its peak, and settle into the afterglow. This is the key. Without it, without the one-pointed attention, it may not work for you.

When you orgasm, you briefly become one with the ocean of energy around you. Your energy field is in touch with this ocean constantly, much as your physical body is in contact with the air around you.

According to the tantric model, the boundaries of your energy field, of your bubble, actually vanish for an instant at the sexual climax. By placing your attention on your energy field and making this whole experience conscious, you have a chance to greatly intensify the sense of oneness and other spiritual intensities of the orgasm. You may also increase the possible healing power, since you are making yourself available to the unlimited energy around you.

Independent of each other, several people capable of intuitively observing the energy field reported to me that during a total let-go orgasm the energy field goes through stages that bear a startling resemblance to the astronomical supernova.

They described how, first, the field swelled and vibrated more rapidly. Then it contracted to a point within the heart. Finally, it expanded in a sudden, blinding flash out from that center point to, apparently, the edges of the universe!

Since red tantra teaches that the universe is the body of the Goddess, is it so surprising that her most fascinating cosmic fireworks display, the supernova, is also the energetic model for a great Fourth of July orgasm?

Naturally, any psychic, energetic or meditative work that you do will contribute to this way of expanding your orgasm. Please be sure to take plenty of time for re-entry after using this technique. Take a long shower. Eat something. Drink plenty of water. When you're ready, ask your partner to do the pleasuring. You should find that this frees up your attention.

If you have a partner who is into this with you, then do the Orgasmic Supernova together. Notice how your fields intermingle and interact. Notice how you are accelerating each other's energy movements, not just your physical reactions.

However, and this is very important, a partner is not at all needed to get the full effect. With or without a partner, this method will expand your orgasmic universe.

At a recent workshop, one of my students, Bill from Seattle, asked "How can this be? When I climax, I'm not there."

I smiled. "That's exactly the point, Bill," I replied. "When you're not there, your freedom, your unbounded identity, is there."

When students start working with the orgasm as a spiritual experience, they think they are doing it. They think they are doing tantra with the orgasm, meditating on the orgasm, but it's the other way around. The orgasm is meditating them. The orgasm is the state of meditation, the ground of being, the blissful pure presence, that tantrikas seek. The orgasm is not just a biological accident, an evolutionary afterthought. The orgasm is where spirit meets flesh, where infinity kisses creation, where the calm, clear, open sky of wisdom embraces the blissful, wild, wet wave of love.

The orgasm is a gift from the higher power, the first-class ticket on a ride that offers every man or woman their fifteen seconds, not of fame, but of timeless mystical wonder.

Trust this most priceless of opportunities, this unique, ecstatic, seductively dancing chance to taste what it is like, what you are like when the small "me" has disappeared and the true, deeper, unlimited self, your secret identity as the universal "I," the one in all, the all in one, has stepped forward from behind the scenes to take its place. The Bible describes the revelation of the orgasm with these words: "I am that I am."

Do you trust the orgasm, nature's wisdom at play, in your body?

Ask yourself this now. It is a most important question. It could be the key to your success at tantra. Though sexual tantra is not just about orgasm, it is in the epiphany of orgasm that the inner light breaks free from the frozen grip of the ego. According to sacred teachings, giving birth, falling asleep, dreaming and dying are also transition states, called *bardos,* in which a gap appears, a white hole in ordinary time and space through which the timeless and infinite may be touched, tasted, listened to, witnessed, felt.

That the orgasm, typically, is brief makes it no less real. Intensity is not measured in clock time. Your sincerity, your eagerness, your earnestness to meet the full moon of your true tantric self face to face is the key. Five seconds of sacred orgasmic surrender could be worth a month of ordinary meditating.

The orgasm is a mini-enlightenment. In the white-hot heat of total fusion with the universe, healing and transformation at the deepest levels are possible. The healing of sexual abuse is, ultimately, a healing of the ability to trust, not just other human beings, but our home, the universe, itself.

This trust grows as understanding deepens. Whatever your story, you are on the same journey with the rest of us. During a sexual climax, you are joining a unified field of consciousness. We are in this together.

A spiritual teacher once said, "I honestly cannot say that 'God is love.' God is a concept and means many things to many people. Some do not believe in God at all. But love is real. We have all experienced love, even if it was just for a moment. In that moment, we felt a truth that made life worth living. So I would say, 'Love is God.'"

In the same spirit, I would like to suggest to you that "Orgasm is God."

In fact, it may open up a new dimension of sexual fulfillment for you—the cosmic climax. In the story, when Jennifer awakens to the spiritual essence of her orgasm, she finds her true self and deep healing at the same time.

TANTRIC TALE

Big Bang

"ARE YOU SURE THIS IS THE RIGHT WAY?" SARA ASKS. IT'S only been twenty minutes since Robert turned the car off the main highway into the forest, but to her it feels like they've been bumping along the unpaved road for hours. On either side of them loom thick walls of pine trees.

"The directions say we'll come to a dirt road," he says. He pauses, and she knows she's pissed him off. "Sara, I have no idea what to expect. I just want to see what it's like. I want to try something different. Ravi just said it was a gathering."

A gathering of perverts, Sara thinks. "It's fine. We're here now."

"It's not an orgy, Sara. He made that clear."

They drive the rest of the way in silence, until they arrive at a house of stone and pine that seems to be made out of the forest itself. As they walk up the wide staircase to the front door, Sara breathes in the crisp evergreen air, willing herself not to be nervous. She is doing this for Robert, she tells herself, to show that she has an open mind. She has to trust him.

Ravi and his wife Chitra, a dark-skinned, almond-eyed woman with long black hair, greet them at the door. Chitra wears a simple red silk sundress so thin that Sara can make out her nipples. Sara feels a twinge of something—fear? excitement?—that she can't identify.

They follow Ravi to a terrace illuminated by yellow lanterns, where four other couples of various ages sip wine and chat in the warm summer night. Ravi steers them to an attractive young couple. The woman, Kirsten, is tall like Sara, with straight, dark blonde hair that falls to her shoulders. A low-cut batik dress cups her slim body. Her boyfriend Anil is tall, slim, and muscular. His wavy black hair brushes against his shoulders, setting off high, wide cheekbones, a dimpled chin and a bright-white smile. As usual when faced with beautiful people, Sara feels both unattractive and un-hip. She looks over Robert. He tucks his long dark hair behind his right ear, a sure sign that he, too, is nervous. Good, she thinks.

"Have you been here before?" Sara asks Kirsten.

"Yes, we have. These are very special evenings." Kirsten's eyes wander around the terrace, and Sara is sure that she would rather be talking to someone else. *We're going to be the couple no one wants to fuck,* Sara thinks, and almost bursts out laughing.

Thankfully, Ravi begins speaking. "Tonight is for pleasure, but it is also for the spirit," he announces. "Tonight we call upon the spirit of Shiva, our divine father, and Shakti, our divine mother, who are always making love, throughout all eternity. May the great Mother Power, the Kundalini, rise up within us and may we surrender to Her, to Her union with Shiva, through each other.

"To facilitate this," he continues, "each couple will have an opportunity to find their own play space in the garden below. The only ground rule for this evening is that you respect each other's privacy and boundaries. May the God and Goddess bless you."

Sara senses someone's eyes on her and looks up to see Anil watching her. Their eyes lock for half a second before Sara, startled, looks away. Her attraction catches her off guard. Since the day she met Robert, she has never been interested in anyone else, and when he tells her that he only has eyes for her, she knows he's telling the truth.

Robert takes her hand, and nuzzles her neck; this public display of attention is another sign that he, too, feels insecure. Did he see the look that passed between her and Anil? She feels the warmth spreading between her legs. She wishes she could make love to Robert right there.

They follow Ravi down a wide stone staircase to the garden. In the center is a raised platform on which stands a large, square bed covered by richly brocaded silk cushions; the perimeter of the garden is made up of numerous, recessed alcoves filled with mats and cushions.

Sara and Robert find themselves standing next to Kirsten and Anil at the entrance to adjacent alcoves. Kirsten turns to them.

"If you would like to join us, please feel free," she says as calmly as a queen.

Sara tries to keep her jaw from dropping. She glances over to Robert and sees that his eyes are wide. She nods and pulls him into their alcove.

Once inside, Sara sees how cleverly the alcoves are designed. The floor, which is flush with the garden floor, is literally padded, like a large, circular bed, and the walls are draped with white muslin that creates a tent-like effect. There are pillows of various shapes and sizes, and a small mahogany table on which sits a plate of fruit and cheese under a cover, several bottles of water, two glasses, condoms, and several white hand towels. Candles flicker in sconces mounted on the walls. Now that she's closer, Sara sees that each alcove is hidden from the one on either side by wooden screens and flowering bushes, and that the ground from their alcove to the center platform rises up gradually but just enough to shield the alcoves opposite them from view.

"Is this all right?" Robert asks as they settle back on the cushions. He pours her a glass of wine. As she drinks it, she feels herself relaxing. She slips her dress over her head with a giggle.

"You could have knocked me over with a feather just now when Kirsten..." Her voice trails off. "Yes, this is beautiful."

"*You* are beautiful." He pauses. "Sweetheart, if you want to go with them, we can. If you don't, I'm fine with that, too."

"What do you want to do?" If he told her that he wanted to go, she knows that she would.

"I want tonight to be our night."

"But you're the one who wanted to come."

As soon as she sees the disappointment on his face, she wants to kick herself. Why can't she keep her mouth shut?

But then, movement on the center platform catches her eye. Illuminated by a hundred candles, Ravi and Chitra have climbed onto the bed and are removing each other's clothes as carefully as if they were unveiling holy relics. Their bodies are not perfect by Western standards—Ravi has the stomach of a Buddha, and Chitra's hips and thighs bear the heavy voluptuousness of a woman who has borne children—but Sara thinks they are the most beautiful couple she has ever seen. They take each other's hands and gaze at each other intently, for several minutes, their chests rising and falling with each breath. Then they begin to kiss tenderly. Chitra moves onto Ravi's lap—Sara sees Ravi's erect penis disappearing into Chitra—and wraps her legs around his waist. They begin to rock together.

Sara looks over at Robert. His eyes are locked on the center platform, and his penis has begun to stir. She leans over and kisses it, then takes it into her mouth and sucks it gently until it hardens. He closes his eyes and moans.

"I love your mouth on me," he says. Then he takes hold of her head. "Come here."

He pulls her to him and kisses her. The air in the garden is thick not only with the smell of star jasmine and plumeria: it has also begun to fill with the perfume of sounds, of sighs, moans, and gentle cries, the tiny, soft collisions of bodies joining. Sara's mind keeps returning to the couple next door. Finally, she pulls back and looks deeply into Robert's eyes. She sees love; she sees acceptance. She gets to her feet and reaches for Robert's hands.

When Robert and Sara come around the screen that separates them, Anil and Kirsten are stretched out naked on the cushions, fondling each other. They look up and smile, then reach out and pull the other couple gently to the cushions. For a moment, all four sit cross-legged, joined by their hands.

Kirsten leans forward and kisses Sara gently on the lips. Sara closes her eyes: She has never kissed a woman before. Her heart races with both curiosity and fear. She allows her mouth to rest on Kirsten's, letting the other woman take the lead and part her lips with her tongue, until at last Sara's tongue responds in kind, even though she still feels only curiosity. Sara feels Kirsten's hand on her breasts. Shyly, she mimics her actions. She has never felt another woman's breasts and is almost surprised by how soft they are. She wonders whether Kirsten will touch her between the legs and whether she will have the courage to touch her back.

But instead she feels hands reach from behind her so that for a moment, there are four hands caressing her breasts. Since she can see Robert, she understands that the hands belong to Anil; she can feel his legs on either side of her, encouraging her to lean back against him. His hands leave Sara's and move down over her rib cage and her stomach. And then lower.

Sara's eyes meet Robert's. He moves behind Kirsten into the same position as Anil, holding Kirsten's torso between his knees. Sara feels as though she is looking into a mirror. At the moment that Robert's hand slips into the golden, curly hair covering Kirsten's sex, Sara feels Anil's finger touch her in the same place. She feels herself swell and knows how wet she must be. As she watches Robert touch Kirsten, Sara realizes that she isn't jealous. She sees that Robert is using Kirsten to show Anil exactly how to touch Sara. *Who is the mirror?* Sara wonders. Anil's fingers imitate Robert's, moving faster and faster against Sara's clitoris. Sara moans and leans back against Anil's chest. She can feel his erection pressing against the small of her back. She unfolds her legs and drapes them over Kirsten's thighs.

She wants to be penetrated. But by whom? It doesn't matter. She feels like a goddess—a magnanimous, beneficent goddess. Her boundaries dissolve.

Anil leans back on the cushion, pulling Sara with him so that her back rests against his smooth chest. Kirsten stretches out with them and continues to tease Sara's nipples. Sara turns her head to Anil so that they can kiss more easily. She throbs under his fingers; she feels close to coming, so she puts her hand on his and slows it.

Robert comes around from behind Kirsten, and Anil moves his hand away so that Robert can cover Sara's sex with his mouth. She gasps as his familiar tongue parts her swollen labia and starts to lick. Behind her, she hears Anil quietly break open a condom wrapper. Then she feels his erection slide down to her wet opening. She has fantasized about being with two men, but has always dismissed the idea as being unworkable. Now, here it is.

"Yes?" Anil whispers in her ear.

"Yes," she gasps.

He enters her, sliding into her slowly, so she can feel every inch of his long, slim penis. She sees that Kirsten has put a condom on Robert and taken him in her mouth, turning her body so that Robert can slide his fingers inside her while she rubs herself. Sara watches Robert make love to Kirsten with his fingers while she masturbates. *Good,* she thinks. She wants to touch her, too. She puts one hand on Kirsten's smooth, golden leg and the other hand on Robert's head, intertwining her fingers in his thick hair. Inside her, Anil begins to thrust—long, hard, deep thrusts that bump against her womb.

Sara's gaze moves to the center platform. Chitra kneels atop Ravi, riding him, her head thrown back so that her long black hair grazes the tops of Ravi's thighs as he caresses her full breasts. Ravi sits up and intertwines his legs with Chitra's. They gaze deeply into each other's eyes, smiling. He takes her face in his hands.

Suddenly, Sara wants only Robert. She reaches down and pulls him up, out of Kirsten's mouth, so that she can kiss him, tasting her own musky smell on his lips. Anil seems to understand, because he pulls out of her, kisses her on the cheek, and goes to Kirsten. Sara watches as they kiss and caress, and as they begin to make love, Sara feels something akin to joy. She turns to Robert and looks into his eyes. Is he all right? But his face is full of love for her. He quickly puts on another condom and slides into her.

"There is no one but you for me," she whispers in his ear. "There will never be anyone but you."

"I know, my love. And you for me."

He moves inside her, his thrusts coming faster and deeper. Around them, from the center platform and the other alcoves, the sounds of love quicken and grow more intense. The current in the night air becomes more concentrated, like a wave forming miles offshore.

Robert slips his hand between their bodies and rubs Sara's clitoris. Already excited, Sara feels the current growing in her belly. She rocks against Robert's fingers like a woman possessed, and just when she thinks she can no longer hold back, she hears ecstatic cries around her and lets herself go. It's not even that she has an orgasm: the orgasm has her, exploding inside her and flinging her into the night sky. She feels Robert come inside her and realizes that they are both crying out, their voices joining in the chorus of pleasure rising up from the circle in the garden.

Finally, their orgasms subside, and she lies in Robert's arms, letting the aftershocks pulse gently through her body. When their breathing returns to normal, they quietly return to their alcove, leaving Anil and Kirsten intertwined. As she and Robert lie down on the cushions, she sees Ravi and Chitra step down from the platform, hand in hand. Chitra catches her eye and smiles. Thus blessed, Sara closes her eyes and dozes.

After a while, the couples in the garden rise one by one, dress, and go into the house. There isn't much talking, but it seems to Sara that everyone glows from within. Sara is relieved that there is no small talk about the future, no exchanging of contact information with empty promises of meeting again. There is only the present. She feels love, and that's enough.

She knows that she and Robert will discuss the evening, but not now. As they bump back down the road, back toward civilization, they give each other the gift of each other's quiet presence, a gift of silence as pregnant as the moment after Creation. This time, the drive passes by all too fast.

TANTRIC EXPERIENCE

Universal Bliss Vibration

TANTRA TEACHES THAT THE SEXUAL ORGASM IS NOT JUST A physical event. In that special moment, there is total unity. Spiritual energy flashes down like lightning into the body through the crown of your head. You achieve a unique experience of unity with the universe because the universe, in that instant, has become one with you.

During sexual orgasm you step effortlessly into the bright, open, infinite state, then in the afterglow, you bask in its brightness. But preconceived ideas about the sexual orgasm can block this total let-go into the enlightened state.

The orgasm is a temporary dropping of the body. If you think the orgasm is just a physical event, the result of brain chemicals mixing together, then you may hold onto the body out of fear. Instead of inviting you to unbounded bliss, the orgasmic surrender will remind you of death. Subconsciously, you will tense up and hold back. The ecstasy of complete bodily surrender, the joy of dissolving into the ocean of life, will escape you.

Tantra says that when the universe flashed into existence, it first created for itself a formless body of pure love and bliss. This Cosmic Body of the Divine Mother lives on, so that a subtle pulsation of bliss is taking place in everything in the universe. The sexual orgasm accesses and downloads this eternal, everywhere present bliss.

Your ecstasy at the orgasm, and then during the afterglow, shows that you have raised your vibration to that of the universal bliss vibration frequency of the universe. You do not create the bliss—the bliss already exists as a universal formless presence. You accelerated your vibration and reached a new, higher frequency, changing your experience.

Tantra uses the metaphor that Shiva, the Divine Father, and Shakti, the Divine Mother, are making love. This universe here is literally the body of the Divine Mother. She and Shiva are making love all of the time, for eternity, and she is in a wide-open, constantly blissful, total let-go state. When you have an orgasm, you are sharing Her orgasmic state. Her bliss is here all the time, always available for your enjoyment.

The afterglow state is a powerful window of opportunity. When you are done climaxing, the fun has just begun. If you pay close attention to the subtleties of the afterglow experience, you will find that an exquisite, healing pleasure that lasts from a few minutes up to half an hour is waiting for you.

During the afterglow stage, you are returning to your physical body from a more expanded place in consciousness. This is true for everybody. But few know about it, and fewer still watch for it. When you watch closely, you will see for yourself that you re-enter body consciousness from a high dimension of vast, shining light.

In the afterglow re-entry journey, you reclaim your physical identity in graduated steps. You start with the wide-open super-bliss space at the peak of the sexual climax. Then you gradually return to everyday body consciousness in waves of pleasure.

Would you like ten or twenty minutes of wonderful whole-body peace and bliss right *after* the ecstasy of your climax? That's a typical afterglow meditation. All you need to do is achieve an orgasm, then lie down and follow this simple secret: Do not move!

Yes, the secret of success with afterglow bliss meditation is stay *completely* still.

You will be able to effortlessly experience the rich nuances of the afterglow re-entry. As you remain in the luminous clarity and blissful spaciousness of the afterglow, you are resting in your natural spiritual state, the essence of your very own beingness. You are meditating in a state of non-effort as you follow this life-giving river of bliss. This is an ancient organic yoga, one of the great secret gifts of mother nature.

Afterglow yoga is best practiced in a tantric meditation asana (yoga position) called Savasana (corpse pose). After you climax, roll onto your back. Just lie there. Don't move. Be relaxed, but try not to even scratch an itch.

If your partner is open to sharing the afterglow space with you, try it as a gentle ending to sessions where one partner pleasures the other. After your partner has brought you to orgasm, just lie back, relax and enjoy the ride back. Since you have no obligations to return the favor in that session, you are free to just be still and fully enjoy the fruits of your sexual yoga, including a leisurely afterglow session.

If you decide to explore afterglow yoga, talk to your partner about it. Otherwise, you may be perceived as being aloof and remote, when in fact you are basking in the pleasure your beloved has bestowed upon you!

A partner once asked me why I wanted to be motionless after having my climax. I replied "You make my body feel so good, I want to relish every moment of it." She smiled with understanding. Still, I kissed, caressed and cuddled her after our ten minutes of afterglow yoga was up, for her wisdom about connecting was right, too!

Here is how you can share the joy of afterglow yoga together. Find a position that you can hold together comfortably for five, ten, even twenty minutes. The spoon position where one partner embraces the other from the back is a good choice. Or perhaps she rests her head on his chest as he lies on his back.

Once you have found your afterglow yoga partner asana, do not move. Relax, soften into the position, and stay completely still. Close your eyes. Feel the flow of energy in your body. Float on your blissful afterglow cloud.

You can definitely share the transcendental afterglow together and enjoy a beautiful, melting fusion, a deepening intimacy after lovemaking. It is like having your cake and eating it, too.

Talking may interfere with this special, expanded space. This is, after all, a meditation. Beautiful music that you both enjoy is fine. Caressing your partner can distract them, too. Caressing is natural at this time. Nonetheless, the moments immediately following the climax are the precious "sweet spot" of the afterglow. If possible, close your eyes within a few seconds of your climax, make your body still and enter your meditation.

If your partner wants contact, kiss them, tell them you love them. Then close your eyes and float in the luminous afterglow flow. Talk to your partner about afterglow meditation *before* you try it. You will not have enough time to explain what you are doing and enter the twenty second afterglow window.

The joy of the afterglow enables deep saturation by the healing rhythms of whole-body rapture. You will be able to hug, cuddle, caress and talk soon enough. This magic window right after sexual climax is the invisible energetic finale. Your physical bodies may be done having sex, but your energy bodies are still dancing, expanding, exploding, flowing, glowing.

Afterglow yoga is a deep yet delicate meditation practice. This is why your eyes are closed and your body is still. After a few afterglow adventures, you will realize that you have been limiting your enjoyment to only the first half of the orgasm cycle.

After the initial rush of the genital climax is over, do savor the subtle thrills of your sacred return to your planetary body. You may be amazed by the almost psychedelic journey in consciousness that is taking place right under your nose after each and every orgasm. There may even be times when your long, slow, sweet hang glide from heaven turns out to be more satisfying than the huffing and puffing up the hill of arousal that got you there.

In the story, Sara and Robert take a spiritual off-road adventure into a luxurious tantric wilderness and discover that there are many paths to the ecstatic, sacred truth of unity. Through their tantra, they realize that all roads eventually lead to the wordless rapture of the Infinite. The blissful, complex playfulness of the Great Mother confounds the mind. Yet She is our home, our source, our beloved, life-giving, pleasure-loving universe. Know your own truth and live it, yet respect and learn from the journeys that others are on.

CHAPTER THREE

Tantric Healing

TANTRIC TALE

Orange Juice

"I'VE LOST MY ORGASM," I TELL JACOB.

"Should we send out a search party?" he answers. He doesn't seem concerned, but I am.

We are lying in his backyard next to the pool, sunning ourselves on towels spread across his lawn. If I lift my head, I can see the glassy aqua surface of the pool, then the fence, and on the other side of the fence the vineyards, stretching down the hill and across the valley, their green branches bending under clusters of grapes. I love it here in the wine country: I love the quiet, the seclusion. Right now, no one can see us except the hawk that flies in lazy circles far above us. So we've left our bathing suits scrunched in a drawer inside Jacob's tiny house behind us. We don't need them.

I've been dating Jacob for three months. We met when I came into his restaurant one night to treat myself after an especially bad day at the boutique where I work. He took one look at my mopey face and brought me a plate of oysters in a saffron-coconut broth with a glass of Chardonnay on the house, and it was love at first bite. Literally. I stayed until the restaurant closed, and then I went home with him. The sex was amazing. It still is.

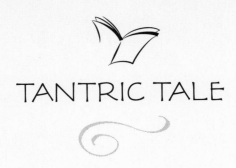

Amazing, except for one problem. I still haven't had an orgasm—the truth is, I've never had an orgasm—and I think he's starting to wonder what's wrong with me. *I'm* certainly wondering what's wrong with me. Jacob is such an amazing lover, I thought for sure he'd be the one to give Tara her first big O. I thought with him, finally, I'd get to find out what everyone was talking about. I thought I'd get to stop obsessing about the fact that at twenty-five, I still hadn't come.

So now I'm glad he's joking, but I'm still embarrassed. I have to take a chance and try to trust him. I roll over and examine a blade of grass. "The problem is, I don't really know what my orgasm looks like."

"So it'll be kind of hard to put its picture on the back of a milk carton."

"Ha ha."

He kisses my shoulder, and I turn my head slightly so he can kiss my lips. Soon we're rolling around on the towel, kissing and fondling. No big surprise there: We can never keep our hands off each other for very long. As our tongues explore each other's mouths, I start to get really excited about the idea of having sex with him out here under the sun. His housemate is at work, so there's no chance of us being surprised by unwanted company. I reach for his penis. But to my surprise, he takes my hands and holds them.

"Sit up." It's an order, not a suggestion. He pulls me to a sitting position. "Cross your legs."

"What? Are you serious?" I examine his thin face closely. I do what he says, but I feel weird sitting there cross-legged and naked.

"You confided in me. Now, I'm going to confide in you. There's part of my life I haven't told you about."

Oh shit. Here it comes. I brace myself for the news that he's married or has another girlfriend. I know he can't be gay—maybe he's bisexual, which I suppose I could handle. He must see the look on my face, because he starts to grin.

"Don't worry. It's nothing bad. But Tara, you have to promise not to laugh."

"I promise."

"You know how I told you I do yoga? I actually do something called Kundalini yoga. And I study tantra."

Relief washes over me, and then, curiosity. "That's cool," I say. "I've been doing Hatha yoga since college. And after I got laid off, I started trying to meditate to deal with the stress. I've heard of kundalini, but I never understood the difference between that and regular yoga. And isn't tantra the one with the one-hour orgasms and all that? I mean, it sounds great, but at this point, I'd be happy with a five-second orgasm."

"It's not just about sex," he replies, laughing. He tells me about tantra, and breath, and the life energy coiled within all of us. He tells me about chakras. It's interesting, and I want to buy it, but I'm not sure what it has to do with my missing orgasm.

"So what does this mean?" I ask when he finally pauses.

"It means I think I know something that might help you. But you have to trust me."

I look at him. In the past, I've gotten in big trouble by trusting men too soon, which is why he's the first person I've let myself date in a year. But something in my gut tells me that this guy is okay.

"I trust you." My eyes feel moist.

He gives me a quick kiss. "Close your eyes and put your hands out in front of you. Palms facing each other."

I feel kind of silly. He tells me to breathe deeply and imagine that I'm holding a ball of energy. This seems kind of abstract, so I pretend that I'm pulling the warmth of the sun down between my palms, where it glows and pulsates. A strange thing happens: My palms actually tingle. Then he tells me to move the ball into the lowest part of my belly, color it bright red, and use it to feed my root chakra, down near my tailbone. I resist the urge to laugh—even though the laughter that bubbles up inside me feels happy rather than mocking—and do as he says. I pretend I'm holding a ball as bright as a fire engine, and I imagine little sparks of electricity shooting down into the area around my butt. I almost feel like bouncing. It's like I just had three double espressos. I'm not jumpy. Just energized.

Then he tells me to imagine that the ball is moving up inside me, but just a little bit, like it's filling my womb.

"Color it orange," he says. "Like a big navel orange of light, expanding out to your sides."

I like this. I picture an orange glow filling my lower body.

"Keep your eyes closed," Jacob whispers. He moves closer to me and pulls me onto his lap, so that my legs are wrapped around him, and his around me. I feel his penis against my opening. I want it inside me, but I can tell he's not going to give it to me yet. He gently touches me between my legs and begins massaging my clitoris with his thumb.

"Breathe, Tara," he says when he hears my gasp of pleasure. "Just let yourself feel it. Enjoy it. Whatever happens, happens."

I picture the ball still pulsing in my womb, streams of energy radiating out from it like a juice as thick as orange honey. I feel unbelievably wet and swollen. Jacob slides into me a tiny bit, rocking my hips with his free hand so that slowly but surely, I rock onto his erection until it fills me. He holds the small of my back with one hand, keeping me close, yet his other hand never loses contact with my clitoris.

"Don't stop imagining the orange energy," he whispers. "And let yourself feel the sensations. Let your body react."

He doesn't have to encourage me any more: My hips begin rocking automatically. His thumb massages me, firmly, intently. I lose track of time. Five minutes? Ten? I don't care. All I care about is the orange ball inside me and the streams of juicy orange honey that are filling my body with warmth. I rock against Jacob's hand.

Then I begin to feel a strange, new, electric sensation, like the orange ball of energy and its streams of light inside me are overflowing into the rest of my body. I'm not sure that I'm controlling the energy anymore; my entire vagina is vibrating. I rub myself against Jacob's hand, and each time I do, I feel him deep inside me. He moves his thumb faster on me, and suddenly, I'm over the edge. This is it, and I can't stop it. And best of all, I know that with him, it's okay.

"Oh my God," I cry as I come for the very first time. Deep inside, I begin pulsing hard around Jacob's penis. Waves of electricity shoot up from my womb and course through my body. Jacob takes his hand away. I don't need it. I'm rubbing and bouncing myself on him like a wild woman. Finally, I collapse against him. A breeze from the vineyard hits us, and I realize that I am covered with sweat.

"I came," I say when I can finally speak. "I came. I don't believe it."

"Believe it," he says in my ear. "Pretty wild, huh?"

I can't let go of him. "I almost feel like I'm still coming."

"So imagine the energy moving through you, up through your body."

I picture the light moving through me from the place where our bodies are still joined, up through my chest, my throat, and finally out the top of my head, toward the cloudless sky. Jacob takes my hands and presses them together.

"This is to ground the energy," he says with a smile. "So it doesn't leak all over the place."

"I think I'm leaking all over you."

We laugh, lie back on the towels, and rearrange ourselves so that we're side by side, my left leg thrown over his slim hip, Jacob still inside me. Our bodies fit each other perfectly. I can feel that he's hard, and I'm amazed. "I thought for sure you'd come, too."

He laughs. "Nah. I was focused on you. Don't get me wrong, it wasn't easy. But it was about you, not me."

These are words I've never heard before from a guy. I look into his gray eyes. And I realize that I've found someone truly special.

"It's your turn," I say, rolling him onto his back so that I'm on top of him. "It's your turn to have a drink of orange juice."

"Only if you promise to share some champagne with me later. I think we need to celebrate."

"Deal," I say, and lower my mouth to his.

TANTRIC EXPERIENCE

Orange Light of Joy

THIS UNIQUE KUNDALINI SEX CHAKRA HEALING MEDITATION enhances sexual response and intensifies orgasmic pleasure for both men and women. It has enabled many women to achieve orgasm for the first time.

To generate the healing power, put your hands in front of you, the palms one foot to two feet apart. Breathe deeply and imagine or feel that energy is building up between your palms. There is an energy center in the middle of each palm.You may feel the results more strongly if you focus there. Breathe deeply and continue to build up energy. Imagine that the energy is taking the shape of a ball, a ball of life-force, of prana or chi. This ball is glowing. It is a powerful, radiant sphere of living light. When you feel that you have done what you can to create the energy ball, place the energy ball into your body at the base of the spine, at the tailbone.

Your energy ball does not have to be perfect. In fact, you may not even be able to feel, see or otherwise sense the energy ball. It doesn't matter. It is still there, and it will still be able to do its job.

Imagine that this energy ball is now centered in your body. Paint it a bright, cheerful cherry red, inside and outside. Continue to breathe into this energy ball. Encourage it to expand and grow in power. Its feeling tone is security and stability.

Now relax and rest in this red energy ball. Instruct it to surround your root chakra and give it nourishment and healing. This red energy ball is now in your body just above the perineum, between the tailbone and the pubic bone. You may get an electrical or charged feeling, like you just plugged into an energy source, which you certainly did!

If you like, you can hold your hands in front of the lower belly, and continue to feed the red energy ball from the centers in your palms. Breathe deeply, gently, and rhythmically. Relax and enjoy. Have fun.

When you feel that you have done all you can do at the root chakra—one to five minutes, depending on how much time you want to take for this meditation—you are ready to move on to the second or sex chakra in front of the sacrum (the triangular bone in your back just above the tailbone). Its color is orange. Its feeling tone is physical joy and the rapture of surrender and fusion.

Now you are in a self-healing rhythm. Breathe deep and pull the big ball of energy at the base of your body up to the second chakra. Allow its color to change from red to orange. Continue to feed it from the front, with your palms in front of your lower belly, if that helps you. Or rest your hands, palms up, on your thighs or in your lap.

Once the orange ball of energy is in place, let it fully surround, embrace, heal, and energize your second chakra. Expect healing and opening there. Allow this center to relax and expand. This chakra can grow bigger, just like a muscle.

In order to encourage the tantric and orgasmic effects of this meditation, continue to feel and concentrate on the orange ball of light, only now encourage it to spread around to the sides of the body, but at the same level. In other words, it doesn't just expand up or down. It spreads sideways so that it is being felt all the way around your body.

You will probably experience that this ball of orange energy is one to two feet in diameter. When you spread the energy around the sides of the body, it will look like a horizontal band of energy. The ball doesn't get bigger. The energy ball retains its integrity, but the living, healing energy that it is radiating gets thicker as it spreads out.

Imagine that the radiation from the orange energy ball is tangible, like golden orange honey or heavy, sweet maple syrup. You are using this warm, thick, juicy, orange-colored life-force to fill up your entire torso in front and around the sex center in the spine. Fill up the body at this level by filling up the front and then the sides. Do this for about five minutes.

This meditation is easy to do because it feels so enjoyable. Sooner or later, you will experience exquisite pleasure. Not only are you clearing out energetic blocks, you are increasing the size and definition of the sex chakra and eliminating negative psychological conditioning.

The bigger the chakra, the better the sexual response. Inability to achieve orgasm or feel pleasure from sexual stimulation shows that the second chakra is not fully opening, not getting excited, not vibrating with rapidity. Once it reaches a state of high excitation, something unexpected happens. It overflows.

It is this overflow of energy that saturates the body and creates undulating waves of pleasure. The bigger the sex center, the bigger the overflow will be, as well as the excitation and the waves. As a result of this volcanic overflow, the pleasure waves cannot stay contained in the chakra, and they engulf the landscape of the body.

Without this overflow, there is a minor climax (or none at all) in the sex center. Like a single match that flares briefly in a metal box, this "genital sneeze" is a spark without a fuel supply. The pleasure is unsatisfying and short-lived.

Doing this meditation improves performance and responsiveness. New neurological and energetic connections boost the effects of sexual stimulation. Ecstatic overflow occurs easily. Erotic fire spreads rapidly through the body, resulting in the pleasurable conflagration of the whole-body orgasm state.

Continue to take the energy up the chakras. The entire meditation exercise is easily completed in twenty minutes, even if you hang out in the first and second chakras for a full five minutes each. The other five chakras (solar plexus, heart, throat, third eye, and crown) will need only one or two minutes each. However, if you just want to do the first two, that's okay.

Sometimes, one of the upper chakras will snag your attention. It may seem to want you to stay longer. It is asking for additional energy in order to heal and balance itself. Stay until a feeling of completion sets in.

The colors for the other chakras are sunshine yellow or bright gold for the third, emerald or apple green for the fourth, deep indigo or smoky blue for the fifth, silver or sky blue for the sixth. If other colors appear in your mind's eye that feel right to you, follow your intuition. Try them out.

When you reach the crown chakra, allow the white-gold kundalini energy to flow out of the crown of your head and down, around, and through your body. This blissful spiritual energy is the descending blessing current of the Divine Mother's universal love energy. It feels wonderful! Let it saturate your body!

When you are done, ground your energy by clasping your hands and pressing the palms of your hands together. Think that you are willing the energy centers at the middle of your palms closed. Say out loud or think to yourself "Disconnect! Disconnect! Disconnect!" or "Close! Close! Close!" You can also accomplish this by pressing your hands against the wall or any natural wooden object (a tree if you are outside). Will the palm centers to close and mentally affirm "Disconnect!" or "Close!"

This flow of energy out of your palm centers happens automatically when you are doing healing, whether it is for yourself or for others. When you are done with a healing session, though, it is crucial that you completely stop this flow.

Otherwise, you will continue to leak life energy out of your hands for hours, even though the session has ended. I found that I was leaking energy from my hands even after talk therapy sessions with clients, so don't think this applies just to spiritual or energy healing. Close your palm centers when you're done!

If you have orgasmic dysfunction, daily practice of the sex chakra charging technique should enable you to achieve orgasms in one to three months. I don't want to offer false hope, but many women have been helped by this inner joy sex center meditation.

The sex center is sensitive to many kinds of shocks. From Chicago, fifty-two-year-old Sarah reported, "I had cobwebs down there! The loss of my husband hit me hard. I thought I would be out of commission forever. Like a vacuum cleaner, it cleared that junk out. When I did make love again, I felt like a virgin!"

You may notice positive results within a week or two. Also, the technique may increase male potency, although this has not been researched. Your sexual well-being will improve according to your individual needs and the level of vitality that you are starting with.

If you do the meditation up through all your chakras, you may also experience enhancement of intuitive, spiritual or healing gifts. If you find that your sex drive has increased, and you need to have more orgasms, or you suddenly are much interested in going out and getting a relationship, this simply means the technique is working!

In the story, Jacob and Tara model for all of us the beauty and benefits of a skillful tantric partnership blessed with a conscious sensitivity to the sex chakra. Though we cannot tell from the ending if they will stay together or stray apart, Jacob's tantric know-how and gentle wisdom made their erotic play wonderfully rewarding, even healing, for both of them.

Pointing to a high place beyond knowledge, the story illustrates the essence of successful tantra, a secret so obvious it is often missed—for all this tantric tech stuff to work, you must be willing to give up enough of the narcissistic ego demand that your focus on your partner brings healing to their heart and supports their greater good and higher being. From this little gift of willingness, all the other miracles, great and small, are born.

TANTRIC TALE

Sexual Healing

IT BEGINS AS A PINPRICK, AS QUICK AND DELICATE AS IF someone has tapped my temple with a sewing needle. If I catch it quickly enough, I can hurry to my bedroom, turn off all the lights, close the curtains, and lie motionless until I'm sure I'm in the clear. If I'm lucky, I'll even fall asleep. But that seldom happens. Usually, once I feel the pinprick, the throbbing isn't far behind. I feel it first at my right temple. Soon, the left will join it, pounding in sympathy, a sister drum. Before long, I won't be able to move my head in either direction without feeling as though someone is impaling my head with a red-hot poker.

My headaches are awesome in their power. And today, I have the king of all headaches.

Dawn, my assistant, comes up behind me, and puts her hands on my shoulders. I know what she's going to say, and I know, too, that she'll send an e-mail to my husband, Randy, warning him.

"You're going home, lady," she tells me. "I can show properties this afternoon."

So I leave the world of lockboxes and mortgages and offers and counter-offers behind, and drive, with difficulty, down Redwood

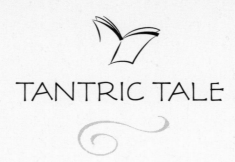

Shores Parkway. Thank God we only live five minutes from my office. At this point, I can barely see. The beautiful, cloudless day, the flowers, the trees, the ducks by the fountain—they might as well not be there. Once I'm inside the house, Allie, our gentle Cocker Spaniel, pads quietly behind me as I make my way down the hallway, touching the walls on either side lightly for support. *Even the dog knows,* comes the thought from somewhere deep in my mind. That's good, I tell myself. I'm still thinking. Sometimes rational thought even stops in the face of this pain. The headache becomes master, and I am just a helpless, useless slave. The more I fight, the worse it becomes.

I strip off my clothes, letting them fall to the floor. Usually, each piece of clothing goes directly from my body to its assigned place in the closet. Not today. I stumble to the bathroom and take some of my headache medication. I might as well be eating a sugar cube for all the good it will do me.

I climb into bed and clutch the pillow over my face. Once I'm horizontal, the pain seems to abate somewhat, like an invading army repelled momentarily. The sheets seem to be trapping the pain against my body, so I kick them off. I try to practice *pranyama,* the deep breathing we learned in the tantra class that Randy and I are taking. For a time, I try to focus on my breath. I even doze.

I wake up when I feel someone sit on the bed.

"Hey, honey-pie. How are you feeling?"

If I were feeling better, Randy's silky voice would be like honey poured over my brain. Now it sounds like he's shouting.

"You look good, anyway," he says. "Really, really good." I remember that I'm completely naked.

I roll over on my stomach. "Go away. Please, honey. Seriously."

He moves to the top of the bed. "Let me massage your temples." He peels the pillow from my head and rolls me onto my back. His fingers stroke my temples lightly, then gradually increase in pressure. He knows just how to touch me. "Breathe," he tells me.

Then he stops and I feel him moving around on the bed. I open my eyes a fraction and notice that he's only wearing his underwear. "You're not getting lucky," I say.

He chuckles. "I'm just going to rub your feet, darling."

Which he does, for what seems like half an hour. Typically, this sends me into heaven—or, if not even, into slumberland. Now it almost seems annoying.

"You don't have to do that," I tell him. "Just hit me over the head with a hammer and knock me out. That's the only thing that's going to help."

He chuckles and slides his hands off my feet to my ankles and calves. I try to imagine I'm getting the world's most fabulous pedicure, and that when I open my eyes, my toes will be painted a lovely, soothing shade of pink. But instead, I feel something wet on my skin. I realize it's his lips.

"What are you doing? Stop that."

He ignores me, and I feel his lips on my inner thigh. I'm feeling about as sexy as a banana slug, and tell him so. But his mouth keeps working his way higher. "Just relax," he says between kisses.

He begins kissing my pubic bone, nuzzling it, and then his tongue begins gently stroking my clitoris. But with the pain in my head, I can hardly feel it.

"Randy, seriously. My head is about to explode."

He lifts his head, smiling. "Shannon, seriously. Just let me do this. If you don't feel anything, I'll stop."

Thus released from the need to perform, I feel myself relax infinitesimally. It's as though the drums in my head suddenly become a fraction quieter.

My will to resist him seeps away.

Randy's tongue flicks my clitoris from side to side, then up and down, the pressure strong, but not insistent. He laps at my vagina, slipping his tongue in and out. In spite of the drumbeat in my head, I sense the first tiny wave of arousal. My hips and legs feel suffused with warmth. A moan escapes my lips, but I'm not sure whether it's from pleasure or pain, because the drums are still there. He moves his tongue up to my clitoris, and, without stopping, slips two fingers into me. I can tell he's curving them to hit the point where my G-spot is supposed to be. I've never believed that I have a G-spot, but what's he's doing feels so good I decide not to worry about it. I just give myself over to the sensation of his tongue on me and his fingers moving slowly in and out.

A single phrase from the *Kama Sutra* floats into my head: "the curve of an elephant's trunk." That's how I imagine Randy's fingers. I push away all judgments—the thought that I must be pretty weird to be thinking about getting fucked by an elephant's trunk has just popped into my brain—and continue to take deep breaths.

And then I have another vision. I am in the jungle, in a clearing, and I am caressing an elephant's trunk. In the distance, drumbeats. Heat presses down on every inch of my skin. I realize that the elephant is gazing at me. I stare back into his endless obsidian eyes, as patient as pools of black sky. I realize that this is Ganesha, ruler of the root chakra, the source of blissful orgasm energy. The energy now radiates from a place deep inside me, a place that Randy seems to be stroking with his fingers. The drums recede into the background, their beat growing fainter and fainter.

As Randy's fingers move inside me, the jungle disappears, and all I can feel is his tongue, stroking me, faster and faster as he senses my approach to orgasm. There's no way I can stop it now. Usually my orgasms start in my toes, but this one starts deep inside my womb, waves of electricity shooting out my fingers and toes like thunderbolts. Randy shows me no mercy. His fingers keep moving inside me, curving against my G-spot, and his tongue keeps caressing me as my hips buck against him. My whole body shakes as the waves of orgasm go on and on, filling my body with warmth.

Finally, my orgasm subsides. Randy lies next to me and strokes my skin lightly, as though he were dispersing the final sparks of energy. He kisses my hair. I realize that my headache is gone. The orgasm has silenced the drums.

"Feel better?" Randy whispers.

"Amazing." It's all I can say. "If you were a doctor, you'd lose your medical license, but that was great."

"I'm in private practice. Very private."

I notice that he has an erection, and I reach inside his shorts. "Can I return the favor?"

"Later." He doesn't push my hand away, but he doesn't move to take things farther, either. He kisses me again, and I sink into the warmth. I fall asleep, my hand still holding his penis, and I begin to dream, once again, of the jungle.

TANTRIC EXPERIENCE

Making Love Is Natural Healing

A FRIEND TOLD ME HE RELIEVED HIS EX-WIFE'S headaches this way. I don't know what exactly he did to bring her to orgasm, but it worked every time. Apparently, she had a lot of headaches.

Sexual arousal to orgasm is a healthy choice. Sex can bring temporary relief to headaches, menstrual pain, and arthritis. Breathing, circulation, strength, and flexibility benefit. The release of endorphins produces the lover's glow, brightening the mood and boosting the immune system.

Tantra says this is just the beginning. Tantra says sex can change your life. Awareness during sex opens the heart. It softens the hearts of men and dissolves their anger. It strengthens the hearts of women and exorcises their fear.

It feeds you what you need.

The essence of tantra is not the fancy ritual technicalities and mystical mumbo-jumbo. The essence of tantra is a profound simplicity: Making love makes more love, brings more love into the world, into your world.

Love, the original wholeness, is always the real healer. This kind of tantra only heals. It will never harm.

In the story, Randy stimulates Shannon's G-spot and clitoris at the same time. I cover this technique in detail in my book *Sexual Energy Ecstasy.* That Shannon's headache went away is based on solid research. Orgasms are good medicine!

Sexual healing is, then, not just healing the sexual part of yourself, but uniting your isolated selves, the lost, lonely, hurt, confused parts, through the magical, mystery power of sexual love. Tantra asserts that you can heal your life with loving sex when that is your conscious intention.

TANTRIC TALE

Natural Beauty

MARIA WALKS. SHE WALKS OUT OF HER HOUSE, GETS INTO her aging Toyota Camry, and drives. She drives away from the rows of tiny houses, their peeling paint, their chain-link fences, their barred windows. *Salsipuedes* is the name of her neighborhood. *Leave if you can.* She drives down a boulevard of endless stoplights, strip malls, and taquerias. She drives towards the hills, past houses whose residents, if they even noticed her, would think she had come to clean.

Maria drives. She drives through a small town of fancy shops and expensive restaurants, full of gifts and food she can't afford, onto a winding road that leads her into the hills. She drives up into the forest, and turns onto the highway that twists along the ridge. Finally, she comes to a parking lot. She pulls into it, gets out, and removes a blanket from the trunk. She takes Juan's gun and puts it in her purse. *There might be mountain lions,* she tells herself. *I saw it in the paper*. Then she sees, in the corner of the trunk, a small box, a box she had almost forgotten. She takes it with her.

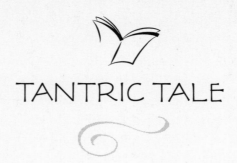

Maria walks onto a hiking trail. The path climbs until she can see the ocean in the distance, then makes a slow descent back into the woods. When she can no longer see the ocean, she leaves the trail and makes her way through the woods. She comes into a clearing. There, she is surprised by a field of sunflowers. Their dark golden heads beckon her. She unfolds the blanket and lays it down at the edge of the clearing. She strips out of the cheap flowered shorts she bought on sale at K-Mart and her thin red T-shirt. *It's okay,* she thinks. *No one can see my bruises here.* She herself now notices them only vaguely—she can't even see the new one on her back, although she knows it's there—but the thought crosses her mind that they are like sunflowers, too, sunflowers of the night. She eases herself back onto the blanket. She takes the gun out of her purse and uses it to anchor a corner of the blanket.

She takes out the small box, opens it, and gazes at the object inside. She thinks of the woman who gave it to her, and the meeting at which she met her.

At the insistence of her friend Lupe, she had attended a women's meeting at the Mexican Cultural Center one night when Juan was out. She took a seat on a folding chair in the back row and sat quietly as words like "empowerment" and "strength" floated over her like bubbles she didn't dare touch. Just as she thought that she, too, would float away and evaporate, she noticed a small, round woman next to her. The woman's presence felt strangely calming. Like an anchor. The woman smiled at Maria, and Maria smiled back. Then the woman took her hand, and Maria, who usually shied away from touch, let her fingers rest in the wrinkled, dry palm.

At the break, the woman handed Maria her card. *Honoria Delgado,* the card said. *Shaman.* Maria had no idea what a shaman was. Honoria smiled.

"Call me," she said.

And Maria did. Honoria poured her coffee and talked to her soothingly. In Honoria's presence, Maria felt calm, safe. Maria told Honoria about Juan. The smell of tequila. The yelling. The money from her paycheck that was always disappearing from her purse.

"You weep for him," Honoria said. "For the sadness inside him."

"Yes," Maria answered, surprised. Her friends and family told her only that Juan was a bad man. "He wasn't always like this."

"I know, little one."

Maria told Honoria about the early days with Juan. She felt herself growing warm as she recounted their lovemaking to the older woman. But Honoria didn't seem embarrassed. She encouraged Maria to talk, and Maria, who had never talked so openly with another woman about sex, found she couldn't stop herself. Finally she paused.

"Do you play with yourself?" Honoria asked.

Maria didn't pause. She wasn't embarrassed."Yes. I can't help it."

"Of course you can't. You are a daughter of the earth. You have found the source of joy. Like the Earth, there are places in you where the water comes out when the right spot is rubbed. This spring is healthy."

Honoria went to her dresser and came back with a box adorned with a mother-of-pearl snake and an eagle inlaid into the box. Maria opened it and saw what looked like a strange mushroom, small at the top, flared toward the middle, then tapering to a curved stem and a flared base. She began to blush.

"Is this . . . is this a, what do you call it . . . a dildo?"

"Yes, child. But this one you put up your ass." Honoria gestured with the little mushroom behind her dress, and Maria laughed. The woman smiled. "First, you take three fingers and make a spiral around your swelling jewel, until you gush from your spring and the cave inside you quakes. When that happens, your sacred power awakens and moves through your flesh."

Maria wasn't sure she understood, but she kept listening.

"When that happens, plant your thumb on yourself and move your fingers inside you. Then put this little one, which is always hard, up your little rosebud and invoke the glory of the Goddess. Call upon your ancestors. It will bring you visions and powers. It will show you truth."

Maria stared at the object in her hand. Honoria continued.

"This is made from the bone of a mountain lion that died defending her cubs," she said. "You are fierce and strong, like that mountain lion. I knew it the first time I saw you."

Maria lies on the blanket. She stares up at the sunflowers. She tries not to look at the gun. Tears form in her eyes and roll down her face, wetting the thick blanket of her hair. Here, where no one can touch her, Maria begins to touch her body in the way that she imagines a lover would. She becomes her own lover, caressing her breasts, rubbing the hard little nubs of her nipples until they jut out stiffly. She rubs her hands over her belly and down over her pubic bone. She has felt nothing in this area for so long that she is afraid nothing will happen, but instead she responds as though a light switch had been flicked on. She swirls three fingers around and around. Her body responds with wetness.

With her other hand, she reaches for the box and pulls out the smooth anal plug. She wets it with her juices and puts it against her tiny, second opening. With her other hand, she does as Honoria told her: She puts her thumb on her clitoris and works three fingers inside herself while, with the other hand, she slowly works the plug into her ass.

She thinks she feels the fingers in her vagina and the finger of bone in her ass touch, and as her thumb presses down, her body convulses with a sharp, metallic kiss of pleasure that radiates from her toes to her breasts to her scalp. Her fingers move in and out on their own, like the tide, in and out, in and out, in and out. Maria closes her eyes and moans, moans to the moon, to her pain:

"Three Sisters, take me home, take me to the Moon, to my mother, to all the daughters and sisters. Please, Three Sisters, read my heart. Ease my pain. Help me. Heal me. Please, Three Sisters. Please."

She doesn't know where these words come from. She offers up her body, her only possession of value, as a sacrifice to the fierce summer sun. She moves her fingers faster and faster.

She feels the sun enter her eyes and kiss her brain. A lava flow of yellow, radiant power suffuses her. She closes her eyes and focuses on the honey-glazed glow at the back of her eyelids.

In the sun, Maria has found her perfect lover: strong, generous, warm. He is not jealous. He does not beat her. He will not lie, cheat, and steal. He will not smell of other women's juices. He will hold her and protect her. She feels the growing heat from his touch.

Maria pulsates with the rhythms of bone, blood, fingers. As her hungry fingers fill her with fire, her thumb dances a spiral on her clitoris, which swells and grows harder and harder in response. Finally,

Maria gives herself over to the orgasm. She is coming, and coming, and coming.

Maria explodes and melts into her great solar lover. He blinds her with brightness. He is inside of her, a supernova that begins within her womb. He is everywhere. He is the death of everything she knows and the bold, bright seed of the new. She floats above the earth and then begins falling and falling, past the cloud cover of her hopes and fears, into the sweet, silent core of her deepest being.

True knowledge erupts from the depths of her womb and spreads through her. True knowledge pours in through every pore, blown in by the heated wind.

She feels like a virgin again. She feels like her own mother. She feels like herself.

A sweet, warm goldenness flows into her. Time and space disappear. This is bliss. This is freedom. Safe at last, Maria falls into a peaceful sleep, a sleep she hasn't known for many, many years.

Maria dreams. Splinters of pain dig deep into her flesh, and a sharp scream chews open her chest. She freezes as if her blood had been replaced by ice. She trembles.

Before her is her bone mother, her Mountain Lion Mother, claws outstretched, her teeth bared. Her snout touches Maria's nose, and her whiskers scrape Maria's face. Maria can smell the blood and death in her mouth.

"Why do you defend your den, Maria?" Mountain Lion Mother rasps. "Abandon your den. Save yourself."

Maria stares at her in confusion and fear.

"A snake lives in your den," says Mountain Lion Mother. "He mates with others. He drinks poison water and maims you with his paws."

Maria begins to cry. "When I try to stand up to him, he brings out his gun and says he's going to kill me."

Tears appear in Mountain Lion Mother's eyes. "I understand. I, too, faced a man's gun. And I died. But I had no choice: I had to defend my cubs. You, Maria, have a choice. You have no cubs yet."

"Are you saying I should leave him?"

Mountain Lion Mother's laugh has the texture of sandpaper.

"Yes! Unless you want to end up like me. You cannot win your fight with him. He lost his own soul when he was a cub, when his father beat him. If you have cubs with him, he will beat them, too, and they will also lose their souls."

"Mother, I feel so lost."

"Ask your heart. It will tell you that hatred is all he knows. Inside, he wants death to release him. His confusion is dark and deep, like the bitter cold of black winter. He will take you with him."

"Yes, Mother." She kisses Mountain Lion Mother on her snout. "I understand."

"When you have cubs, Maria, be kind to them. But now, you must be kind to yourself."

Mountain Lion Mother's voice fades until the only sound is of the warm wind rustling through the sunflowers. Maria wakes, opens her eyes, and stands up. She stretches her arms wide. She tingles with new energy.

"Thank you," she says to the world around her. She feels the truth of the words in her flesh.

Her eyes alight on the gun. She kneels at the edge of the blanket, and begins to dig with her bare hands. When the hole is deep enough, she wraps the blanket around her hand and pushes the gun into its soft, brown grave.

Maria drives. She drives down the winding ridge road, down the mountain, and out of the forest. The gun lies beneath the dirt, at the edge of the field of sunflowers. Almost automatically, Maria begins to turn onto the road that will take her back to her husband's house. But then a single word bursts into her brain.

No.

"No!" she screams into the wind. "No, no, no!"

Maria turns the car and drives toward Honoria's house, not to stay, but as a starting place for her new journey, her solo journey. She offers a prayer to the wind. She asks it to carry her "no" to Mountain Lion Mother, so that she, too, will find peace.

Maria drives. She drives toward shelter. She drives toward love. She drives toward her self.

TANTRIC EXPERIENCE

Be Vulnerable to Beauty

TWO FANTASTIC TIBETAN MONKS, THE KHENPO BROTHERS, live in New York City. They are surely enlightened, if anyone is. I had the great good fortune to hear them talk on the topic of "how to love." They revealed a great tantric secret that night.

"People see ugliness in themselves and each other and then struggle to love that ugliness," they said. "That will never work. Instead, dwell on the beauty you see, on even the tiniest positive. Love will flow naturally and effortlessly. It is the nature of beauty to draw out love like a magnet."

Gazing at their radiant, smiling faces, I had no doubt that they lived every word of their teaching.

Instead of fighting ugliness, embrace beauty. Beauty opens and expands whatever it touches. This is the miracle power of beauty, an invisible, irresistible force that initiates the movement to love.

Maria achieved her awakening of courage by celebrating the natural beauty in and around her body. In my workshops, we do a related and less dramatic process with teddy bears. It amazes me how quickly students fall in love with their soft, safe, beautiful teddy bears. It amuses me when they realize that this means they have the ability to love anyone and anything without conditions. Now what will they do?

Maria merged with nature using a sacred personal power object. You can use your anal vibrator or anal plug to claim your power in a similar way.

Tantra must be done with great sensitivity, like Maria in the story. If you do tantra as a technique, in a mechanical way, then you will stay on the surface. You will get mechanical results.

Merger requires opening and penetration. Union with the beloved—a person, a teddy bear, a crystal dildo, the sun in the sky—means you are giving them permission to open you up, to wound you if necessary. This is the definition of vulnerability. Your willingness to allow your love object to wound you creates the opening. You trust them that much.

In the story, Maria is willing to let a wise, aggressive force, Mountain Lion Mother, teach her. She is in denial. She is blind to the evil in her home. She needs a compassionate shock. Maria needs tough love.

The wound inflicted by the beloved is a gift. Like the grain of sand that irritates the clam shell into crafting a beautiful pearl, the wound of love absorbs the magnetic charm of the outer beauty to turn on the inner electrical current of your inborn radiance.

Sexual energy creates life. It created your body. Conscious sex can help give birth to the new forms you need in your life now. If you think you may be frozen by a fear of getting hurt, ask yourself these questions about your life: Where am I putting most of my energy? Am I putting more energy into pushing away what I don't want? Or am I putting more energy into moving towards what I do want?

In spite of all the confusion that surrounds tantra today, there is, nonetheless, a one word definition for tantra. That word is "Yes!"

For all of its complexity, life at every level has only two movements: moving towards and moving away from something. You breathe in. You breathe out. You accept. You reject. You move towards and embrace. You hold back and turn away.

Yes.

No.

When you hold back, it's like holding your breath. For all you know, you could be putting your whole life on hold.

Let life breathe you.

Trust that when you breathe out, life will fill you with fresh life force, with exciting, new, expanding experiences.

Say "Yes!" to life. Maria did.

TANTRIC TALE

Spank Me, Thank Me

I HAD JUST FINISHED PUTTING THE GRANDKIDS TO BED WHEN Bob called to me from the study. I tiptoed down the hallway and found him standing in front of the bookshelves, grinning. He was holding a book, and as I walked toward him, he made a big show of hiding it behind his back. But I could see what it was: *The New Joy of Sex*.

I raised my eyebrows at him. We have a standing agreement that when we babysit for Deb and Scott, we'll resist our parental urge to be nosy, so I didn't approve of him poking through their library, and he knew it.

"What've you got there, Grandpa?"

He flashed a few pages at me. Black-and-white drawings of couples in various sexual positions jumped out at me.

"Oh, for Pete's sake," I said. "I don't want to know my daughter's reading sex manuals. Put that away this second and let's go watch our movie."

But when Bob came into the living room, I saw that he still had the book in his hand. He winked at me as he slipped it into my tote bag.

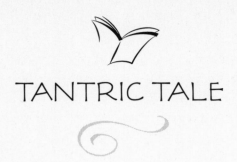

"Don't worry. I'll give it back."

"What if they notice?"

"If they say anything, I'll confess. But I bet they won't."

But I couldn't concentrate on the movie on television. I couldn't forget that inside my innocent canvas tote bag, with its cheerful needlepoint sailboats and seagulls, was a book depicting couples performing every kind of sexual act.

When Deb and Scott finally did come home, I felt like I was blushing as I described what the children ate, what they did, how many times they went potty, and what they did at bedtime. All I could think of was those black-and-white pictures. I kept forgetting things and stumbling over my words. I could hardly wait to get out of there.

Driving away from their house, I was seventeen again and leaving on a date with Bob, all the while knowing that our destination wasn't the sock hop but actually Inspiration Point, and that instead of drinking punch in the church social hall and dancing the Jitterbug, we'd be guzzling beer and doing everything we could think of short of losing our virginity. I remembered how guilty I felt kissing my mom goodbye when my mind was on how soon I could get my hands down Bob's pants. I began to laugh.

"I haven't heard that giggle in a while," Bob said.

"I was thinking about Inspiration Point."

"Oh," was all he said. "Oh." He kept his eyes on the road. After forty years with the man, his silence didn't bother me anymore. Eventually, he always told me what he was thinking.

When we got home, I decided to take a little more care than usual getting ready for bed. I put on the red satin nightgown Bob bought me for Valentine's Day, rubbed his favorite lotion into my skin, and took my hair down. Then I looked at myself in the mirror. I was a little heavy around the tummy and hips, but I didn't care: Bob had always loved my curves. I peered at my face, but things were in pretty good shape. I gave my image a coy smile. *You silly old bag,* I told myself affectionately. *Go out there and seduce your husband.*

But when I came out of the bathroom, Bob was sitting on the bed in just his pajama bottoms, the book next to him. He wore a dejected look on his face, and he slumped slightly, letting the flesh of his belly roll over his waistband.

"Carol, I feel very guilty about taking this book," he told me.

"Well, if you feel that badly about it, I can take it back tomorrow while the kids are at work. They'll never know."

"No, Carol. That's not enough."

I looked at him closely. "What are you talking about?"

"I need to be punished."

I suddenly felt a little lightheaded, so I sat down on the bed next to him. "You do?"

"Yes, Carol, I do. I need to be punished."

I stared at him. Seeing that I wasn't getting his point—whatever it was—he tilted his head to the side, indicating the book. I gingerly turned it over and saw that it was open to a page showing a man about to administer a sound slap to a woman's bum. Maybe this was one of his jokes, I thought. Well, I could play along.

"Punished. Yes. You've been a very, very bad boy." I spoke in a voice I hadn't used for more than twenty-five years. "You certainly have to be punished before you can have any *treats*." To emphasize the last word, I ran my hands over the red satin covering my breasts.

I saw from the expression on his face that he was trying not to laugh—as was I—but I also noticed that a bulge was growing in his pajamas. I picked up the book and studied it long enough to get a few ideas. I stood up.

"What are you going to do?" Bob asked. His tone was both nervous and excited.

"First, you have to call me 'ma'am' until I say you can stop."

"Yes, ma'am."

"Very good. Now, take your pants off and lie down on the bed."

He eagerly slipped off his pajama bottoms and I saw, much to my surprise, that he was completely hard. There'd be no need for Viagra that night!

I pointed to his penis. "That is very bad. I might have to punish you a little more for that. Now, lie down."

"Yes, ma'am." He lay down on the bed.

"What kind of punishment do you think you deserve?"

"A spanking, ma'am" he whispered.

I was surprised. We hadn't spanked our kids—just a swat on the butt now and then to get their attention. My parents had done the same with me, and I certainly never felt abused. But Bob's experience had been different. He joked about the whackings his parents had given him, especially his mother, but I could always tell how painful these memories were. Why in the world would he want to be spanked now?

"Are you sure?" I asked him. I kept my tone severe.

"Yes, ma'am," he said, his voice muffled by a pillow.

Well, he was a big boy. If that's what he wanted, that's what he'd get. I knelt on the floor beside him and put my lips to his ear. "How many spanks do you think you deserve?"

"Ten. No, twenty. Ma'am."

"Twenty! Have you really been that bad?"

"Yup. I mean, yes, ma'am."

"All right then."

Climbing onto the bed next to him, I knelt by his side. I looked at his poor ass cheeks. They seemed to quiver slightly. Could I really do this? Even though we'd had some awfully big fights over the years—you can't be married as long as we have without some big disagreements—I had never even thought of raising a hand to Bob. I took a deep breath. "Are you ready?"

"Yes, ma'am."

Just as I raised my hand, I had a moment of uncertainty. What if I was doing this wrong? I quietly stole a glance at the book. "Uh, Bob?"

"Yes ma'am?"

"How will I know if what I'm doing is too much?"

"I'll say the word 'silver,' ma'am."

"Good. Be sure you use it. Don't try to be macho."

"Yes, ma'am."

I took a deep breath and then brought my hand down on Bob's butt. He hardly reacted other than to say, "One. Thank you, ma'am."

His voice startled me. Why was he talking? I glanced over at the book.

"It's okay, Carol," came Bob's muffled voice from the pillow. "I saw it in a movie."

What movie? I wanted to ask him, but I didn't want to break the mood. However, the thought of him watching dirty movies without me—well, I can't say it outraged me, exactly, but it definitely irritated me. I brought my hand down on his butt a little harder than before. This time, he jumped a little.

"Two. Thank you, ma'am."

"Did I give you permission to watch movies like that? I don't think I did!" Whack!

"Three. Thank you, ma'am."

I can't say that I enjoyed spanking him—I was too worried about hurting him—but I guess I was, as our kids would say, "getting into it." I decided to pretend I was just acting another role, like the high school plays in which I'd starred so many years ago. I made the next spank even harder. Whack!

"Four. Thank you, ma'am."

As I continued to paddle Bob, his butt cheeks began to turn a fine shade of cherry red. I kept waiting to hear 'silver,' but I didn't. Instead, when Bob counted his tenth spank, I heard a catch in his throat, a choking sound I hadn't heard since the birth of our children. Was Bob crying? Suddenly, I was terrified. Maybe I'd gone too far.

"Honey, are you okay?" I said, leaning forward.

"Yes, ma'am. Please continue."

"Are you sure?"

"Yes, ma'am. Please continue."

You could have knocked me over with a feather, I was so surprised. But I thought to myself again, *He's a big boy. If this is what he wants, I'll give it to him.* Whack! Eleven. Twelve. I watched him carefully. If he started sobbing, I would stop, but his voice only got more quiet and dreamy, like he was in a trance. If I hadn't known better, I would have said he was stoned. But Bob never let anything stronger than alcohol pass his lips. Whack!

Then I started to notice something. I had an urge to touch myself—something I'd never done in front of Bob. But with his face pressed into the pillow, I knew he couldn't see me. I pushed up my nightgown and slipped my fingers between my legs. Whack! With each spank, I got more turned on. In fact, I was getting wet. Eighteen, nineteen, twenty.

"Twenty. Thank you, ma'am."

I fell down onto the bed beside Bob and rolled him over. I saw immediately that his eyes were wet, and yet he was smiling.

"Honey, are you okay?"

"Okay? I'm more than okay. That hurt like hell. Get on top of me, woman!"

I looked down to see his erect penis pointing straight toward the ceiling. I was wet, but just to make sure, I grabbed the K-Y from our bedside drawer and quickly put some on both of us. He pulled me on top of him and began thrusting as though his life depended on it. I kept watching his face for signs of hurt and anger, but there were none: His smile stretched from ear to ear. He squeezed my breasts, tweaked my nipples, and ran his hands over my hips and bottom. It felt so good, I decided *What the hell* and moved my hand back between my legs.

"Do you mind if I do this?"

His eyes lit up.

"Are you kidding?"

As I rubbed myself, I moved faster and faster on Bob. Suddenly, I felt his hand on mine.

"Show me how to do that."

I took his fingers and put them in the right place. With both our fingers moving together, the pressure was just right. I felt the tingling begin deep inside me. My eyes flew open as the waves of pleasure raced through my body. I threw back my head and moaned.

"Oh my God, Bob, I'm coming!"

Bob let himself go, too, and together, we bucked and thrashed on the bed. We held onto each other for dear life as our orgasms shook us.

Afterwards, as we lay on the bed, Bob pulled me close. "Do you know how beautiful you are to me?" he whispered, kissing my forehead.

"Did I hurt you, dear?"

"No. It was incredible. At one point, I felt like crying. I was embarrassed. But then that passed and my whole body began tingling. Like I was waking up under a cold shower after a long sleep." He raised himself onto one elbow and looked down at me.

"You know, Carol, there are times when I've felt guilty about our lovemaking."

"Guilty? What on earth for?"

"It wasn't until you mentioned Inspiration Point that I realized why. I always felt that we were doing something bad. I kept waiting for my parents to barge into the room and tan my hide. But I didn't feel that way just now. I think it was because I got punished *before* we had sex! And it was great!"

"That's the craziest thing I've ever heard!"

"Hell, I know! But it worked!" He raised an eyebrow. "Now, don't get the idea that you get to spank me all the time."

"Only if you're very, very bad."

He chuckled and leaned in to kiss me. My foot bumped against the book at the end of the bed, and I gently pushed it to the floor. We wouldn't need it again.

Tantric S&M

WHAT IS "TANTRIC S&M"? THE EASY ANSWER, OF course, is S&M approached in a tantric way, or performed with a tantric flavor. S&M is itself an unfortunate label. Originally, it was an abbreviation for sadism and masochism, judgmental labels taken from outdated styles of psychiatry.

I think it's more useful to think of S&M as D&S—dominance and submission—combined with B&D—bondage and discipline. What this alphabet soup refers to is something we all understand to some extent from everyday life: the exchange of power. However, I will use S&M here because it is still the most popular label.

In *The Happy Hooker,* creative yet sophisticated call girl Xaviera Hollander describes famous politicians and other men of power coming to her and wishing to be spanked, fed by bottle, and otherwise treated like babies. The extreme yang of being a domineering leader is flipped over to the extreme yin of being a helpless, irresponsible adult baby. As bizarre as this seems, it was healthy and balancing for these individuals.

The Tao does not move in a linear way. It flip-flops from yang to yin and vice versa whenever the energy in one form reaches a maximum or crisis point. The sexual climax is just such a crisis or climax of energy. Most people will find exploring both Top and Bottom roles quite rewarding. Both roles offer unique pleasures, discoveries, and rewards.

The famous Gestalt psychologist Fritz Perls often characterized human interactions as taking place between a Top Dog person and a Bottom Dog person. He observed that in real life, these roles easily reverse.

S&M sex is sex from the third chakra, the chakra of power with, over, under, and through other people. The third chakra is the interpersonal power or social pecking-order center. It is concerned with rituals, rules, roles, and status, with clearly defining who is Top Dog and who is Bottom Dog. Though the third chakra, associated with the solar plexus, is "higher" in the sense that it deals with a broader spectrum of life and issues, with your place in society as a whole, it is not superior to the lower two chakras.

S&M is a sexually sophisticated study of conflict, duality, and power dynamics. This makes S&M a good study for tantrikas who hide behind weakness, niceness, and passivity; then tantric "surrender" tends to be compromise, a way to stay safe and protect a weak ego. The real-world power games of S&M can bring "tough love" healing to tantrikas ready to stop being victims and embrace the personal power stored in their dark side.

What I discovered from dabbling in this area—I do not claim to be an expert, but I was lucky to have good teachers—is that there are two kinds of S&M: traditional and spiritual. Within the domain of spiritual S&M, there are also two popular expressions—the shamanic and the tantric paths.

In conventional S&M, extreme stimulation is used to bring about a state of intensified release for the Bottom, the so-called "masochistic" half of the D&S equation. For his or her efforts, the Top or "sadistic" half gets the reward of doing their job well. Having topped as well as bottomed, I can assure you that the glory of being dominant and appearing to have control over the very soul of another human being is grossly overrated.

The Top does all the work! He or she has to prepare everything, set up all the toys and supplies and make sure that it all goes well so that the Bottom does not get hurt. Remember, S&M is about "safe play." When it crosses that line and permanent damage results, then it is neither safe nor play. Done properly, S&M techniques intensify sexual and emotional release. They also promote and deepen the bond between play partners.

In doing spiritual S&M, we choose between the shamanic approach and the tantric style. In shamanism, the goal is to leave the body. The shaman intends to return, as this is not a method of suicide. Based on my research, profound disassociation from the body is key to the shamanic approach. The shaman travels to other worlds and brings back a valuable message.

Both approaches have as their goal attaining high altered states safely and naturally, but tantra does not emphasize disassociation. Instead, it emphasizes awakening the kundalini within the body and allowing this energy to rise, circulate in the body, and uplift the consciousness.

In tantra, you begin by surrendering to your partner as Shiva or Shakti, but you do not end there. You must graduate to surrendering to the Divine Mother Power within you—the kundalini. When awakened, it may be felt as heat, currents of energy, electricity or other energetic expressions. Or you may just feel bliss, openness, peace.

Do not merely surrender to your partner. If you stop there, perhaps you are feeling love, but tantra says goes further. See beyond their personality to the archetype, the supreme self, they represent. Tantra is erotic love plus meditative surrender plus the union of opposites plus the sacred unknown, a Cosmic X Force that is the sudden lightning strike of enlightenment, the paradox of duality dissolved.

How does S&M help to liberate this mysterious force of nature, the Mother Kundalini?

Often, the kundalini is activated by a sudden life crisis of some kind. Any sort of stress—it could be physical, emotional, mental, spiritual, circumstantial—can precipitate the awakening of this internal power. Like the classic urban folktale of the mother who suddenly gains superhuman strength and lifts a car to rescue her child, in times of great stress, the Power Within steps forward to help people deal with seemingly impossible challenges.

Tantric S&M intentionally creates and applies a carefully controlled physical stress as a sexospiritual discipline. There needs to be considerable trust between the partners. However, at least at the level of a little spanking, tantric S&M need not be expensive, explosive or dangerous. It can be good, cheap, high-octane fun!

How exactly do you go about conscious spanking? And if you choose to do this, how do you make it specifically tantric?

Let's keep it simple, safe, and easy. The first session will be limited to thirty spanks. That's all. If that sounds like too many, then reduce that number to twenty, or even ten. Who makes this decision? The Receiver or Bottom role-playing person takes that responsibility.

Whatever the Top says is, at best, just a recommendation. The Bottom must know herself or himself well enough to gauge what she can handle and can't handle—or is in the mood for that day.

If ten spanks is all you want for your first session, or any session, then that's it. You are the Boss, not the Top. It is your body.

The Bottom lies on the bed, couch or Top's lap with his or her rear exposed. Obviously, you can dress this ritual up as much as you want and ease into it. You can dine by candlelight and dance first. You can spank to the jamming funk of "Give It to Me Baby" by Rick James (which has a distinctive spanking or slapping sound accenting the beat).

The Top says, "Are you ready to receive your spanking?" (Or ". . . your punishment?" This depends on whether or not the notion of getting punished inspires deeper release for the Bottom). If the Bottom is ready, she says "Yes, Master" if the Top is a man. If the Top is a woman, then she is respectfully addressed with the phrase "Yes, Mistress."

The Top administers one spank to each buttock using the open palm of his hand. He makes this spank moderate. It is not light. It is not heavy. It should sting the Bottom a little. It should leave a slight redness where the spank was delivered.

The Bottom will say "One. Thank you, Master." Then "Two. Thank you, Master."

Here, the Bottom has done two things correctly. First, she has counted the spank. Second, she has acknowledged the presence and responsibilities of the Top.

While these ritualistic precautions are of greater significance when the stimulation strategy is more extreme, this structure is proper S&M. In contrast to conventional sexual behavior, S&M sex is clearly defined and intentionally designed. Vanilla lovers can learn a lot from the care and attention to detail that is built into a good S&M session.

Now the Top proceeds to perform all the spanks that were negotiated and agreed to prior to the session. That means this negotiation took place long before the foreplay stage. Both partners were fully clothed and in a normal state of mind. Again, these precautions apply more to extreme scenes, but these principles are basic to all healthy S&M experiences. Specifically, drugs and alcohol have absolutely *no* place in tantric S&M. Do not even think about it!

As the Top proceeds to administer the spanks—exactly the negotiated number, no more and no less—he or she will increase the intensity of the spanks. This is expected. Also, the Top will "mix it up" so that the Bottom is not certain what to expect next.

This brings up the mother of all S&M questions: How exactly does the Top know how much is just enough and how much is too much?

The answer is the Safe Word. During the session the Bottom may make statements like "Oh, shit, that hurts!" Or "Please stop. Please. I can't stand the pain." Or "You call yourself a Top? You're a total wimp!" Since it is completely impossible for the Top to know what the Bottom is going through from statements like these, a Safe Word is agreed to before the session.

The Safe Word is a word that would ordinarily never end up in an S&M session—"banana," for example. Long before your session starts, pick a fun, colorful word you both want to use. It just can't be one that you might spontaneously say under those circumstances, such as "God" or "Help" or "Shit."

If the Bottom says the Safe Word, then the Top immediately stops and attends to the needs of the Bottom. The session is over. The Top addresses the needs of the Bottom, whether they are physical, emotional, mental or spiritual.

Assuming that the session is finished without the Safe Word being uttered, which should be the usual situation, then after the last spank the Top rubs and soothes the Bottom's burning buttocks and otherwise does what he or she can for the Bottom. For example, the Bottom may want to be held by the Top. Or the Bottom may want to have soothing salve applied to her reddened bottom.

Believe it or not, you are still just doing a conventional S&M spanking session. Most people stop here. You do not have to stop here. The key to bringing a spiritual element into an action as mundane, even crude, as spanking is intention. In fact, intention is the core of spiritual practice regardless of how it looks from the outside.

Sitting meditation, for example, transcends mere sitting. Although a good, firm posture is helpful, you can slouch on the couch and meditate if first you set your intention to make that "asana"—the couch slouching position—a spiritual practice. If you don't believe me, then try it. Likewise, walking, eating, and drinking can be transformed through the power of a clear, dedicated intention. Mental attitude transcends bodily position or physical activity.

The first step in making S&M spanking tantric, then, is to have the clear intention that you are doing this to awaken spiritual consciousness in each other. This practice might in some way, perhaps unexpected, benefit both of you.

One of the little-known secrets of the spiritual path is that you tend to learn more from pain than pleasure. Not that it has to be that way. But because society is so confused about the true nature of pleasure and its relationship to higher states and the deep self, you are left with learning through pain until, somehow, you figure out how to learn from your pleasurable experiences as well. Pain has a sharp, demanding edge that helps to keep you alert, while pleasure serves up a dreamy, seductive sensual massage that encourages fuzziness.

In a tantric spanking session, sex, which is pleasurable, is combined in a safe, intentional, and structured way with physical punishment, which is painful. Through the juxtaposition of these two opposites, some kind of breakthrough, some sort of insight, some degree of release, takes place.

Though the Top does not have the advantage of a meditation object like strong physical sensation, the Top must perform his or her duties with mindfulness and compassion. This makes the Top's actions a meditation, too.

The person in the Bottom role is the one feeling the pain, so they are more likely to achieve the breakthrough. This is why I recommend that you switch roles. Both need to Top as well as Bottom. If either of you is tired, then wait until another day to play and exchange roles.

Let's say you are the Top and I am the Bottom. As you spank me in this slow, intentional, structured way, I focus my entire attention on that area of my body, on my buttocks. I allow myself to enter into this area and fully feel it. Further, I allow the sensations and the echoes of those sensations to vibrate and deeply resonate throughout my entire body, to every extremity, and through the entire body as a unified whole. It is like my body is a human musical instrument and it is being played, albeit a little roughly.

Do you understand what is going on here? I am transforming the apparent "poison" of the pain you are creating in my body into the "nectar" of a more awakened awareness of and sensitivity to my body. I may find that certain areas resist, while others yield. I may find that early memories surface to be surrendered. I may find myself having an energy orgasm without any overtly sexual stimulation due to the whole-body energy arousal created by this method. Pain promotes a highly workable state of vivid awareness suitable for meditation.

Also, after such a spanking session, I may be more opened up. This might be especially noticeable to me, even you, if we actually go ahead and make love right after. This is by no means expected or part of the process officially. But if I were seeking to be more vulnerable and available during lovemaking, then being the Bottom and surrendering to the loving discipline of my Top might be a great way to prepare.

What makes spanking tantric? Turning pain into a meditation. Whether we like it or not, pain grabs and holds our attention in a way that pleasure, with its light, frivolous, playful personality, usually does not.

The exception is the higher levels of bliss achieved in sexual tantra and classic meditations like kundalini and anapanasati (following the breath). These bliss states are more powerful and focused than pain is, but this must be realized through practice.

Ironically, when you work through pain via deep meditation, you discover that most of your suffering around pain is simply your fear of it. As your fear of pain dissolves, your capacity to open to all pleasure deepens. Over time, embracing pain consciously and intentionally turns into skillful means, reliably helping you to achieve your goal of rich, deeply fulfilling pleasure.

In the story, Bob and Carol suddenly rekindle sexual desire when they spontaneously embrace Bob's negative childhood memories. A willingness to explore the subtleties of sexual guilt and shame reaps a delightful erotic reward.

S&M practices are not only for the leather facemask crowd. For sweethearts Bob and Carol, their long-time love goes from sugar sweet to spicy hot. They demonstrate that the "thank you" you utter when your lover spanks you may just be the start of the lusty, burning love you both secretly want.

CHAPTER FOUR

Tantric Touching

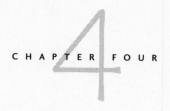

TANTRIC TALE

Heart Center

JOSEPH HAS TO WAIT UNTIL ALMOST NINE O'CLOCK BEFORE his last coworker goes home and he can read the e-mail from his sister in privacy. Just to be sure he's finally alone, he eases up in his chair and looks over the wall of his cubicle. His company's offices are lodged in a former mattress factory converted to loft space; when it's empty, as it is now, it's as silent as a cathedral. He glimpses the lights of the city through the windows that stretch all the way to the top of the two-story space. He sinks back into his chair, back into his fabric-lined cell.

He closes the program he's been working on and re-opens the e-mail. *Maybe this Web site will help your love life,* Amy's message says. *It couldn't hurt, anyway.* He clicks on the link. An amateurish Web page, clearly created by someone who has only recently learned Web design, appears on the screen, and Joseph realizes instantly that the site belongs to a meditation center. "Open Your Heart," a large headline tells him in large type, but instead of opening, his heart plummets. He should have known. Leave it to his kooky sister to think that sitting around with a bunch of woo-woos was going to get him a date.

His eyes fall on another headline that says "Begin your journey on the path of ecstasy," and below it, in blue letters, are the words "The Path of Tantra." Tantra? From the distant past comes a memory of the *Kama Sutra*. He has a vision of long-legged Sharon in marketing, her legs wrapped around him in an impossible position.

Joseph begins to read. When he next looks at the clock, it's two A.M., and he feels like he's been given the keys to the universe.

Joseph stands in the middle of his tiny studio. Suddenly, it appears cluttered and dirty to him. The energy is wrong, he thinks, surprising himself. He's not a guy who's ever thought of a room's "energy." He looks at the putty-colored walls. Tomorrow he'll paint them, he decides. Maybe he'll paint them red. He pulls out a box and begins to throw things in it: clothes he never wears, computer manuals, broken pieces of electronic equipment. At some point, he stops. He looks out his one window at the lights of the city in the distance. Exhaustion sweeps over him, but he's not ready for sleep yet.

Joseph takes off his clothes, crawls into bed and thinks about the technique described on the Web site. He makes an "O" of his thumb and third finger, his tried-and-true hand position for masturbating, and then begins to stroke himself until the sheets tent around him. At first, he imagines Sharon, but somehow, that doesn't seem right, so he focuses on the feeling of his shaft under his fingers. Before long, he realizes he's close to coming. He slows down, remembering the site's words: *Bring yourself to the edge, and then back off*. It's excruciating at first, but soon he turns it into a game to see how close he can get: once, twice, three times. Then he imagines a tube—the Alaskan pipeline!—pumping golden oil between his penis and his heart. The image sends Joseph coursing toward orgasm, and he puts his hand on his chest. He lets go, his hips bucking against the bed. And then he melts into the sheets.

Over the next month, Joseph fills his studio—or doesn't fill it, because he finds that he prefers to have as little clutter as possible—with sleek, dark, cushioned furniture. At work, he counts the hours until everyone goes home and he can go back to the Web site. It becomes his guide, his guru: every night it gives him a new revelation. He learns about chakras and *bardos* and energy. He learns about his heart. And when his eyes become blurry from reading, he goes home to open up that golden pipeline between his penis and his heart.

Sometimes, before he goes to bed, he turns on his computer and visits the Web site once again. But usually he confines his reading to those quiet after-work hours in the brick loft. It is his church. His home is where he puts what he learns into practice, thrashing and writhing on the sheets. His monk's cell.

One Saturday morning a few months later, Joseph realizes that his entire world has been confined to his office and his apartment, with occasional trips to the grocery store and the gym. He goes to the café on the corner, and sits on a bench outside with his coffee, the morning sun warming his face.

An older woman sits down on the bench next him. She has short, gray hair and a wide, tanned face, and she wears a simple denim shirt, khaki pants, and running shoes. When she catches Joseph looking at her, she smiles.

"Good morning," she says. "You look happy."

"I do? I guess it's nice to be outside."

"You spend a lot of time indoors?"

"Yeah. I'm a computer programmer. You look tan. What do you do?"

"I'm a nun."

He stares at her. "You're kidding. I thought . . ."

"You thought nuns stayed inside the convent all day, saying rosaries? Some of us follow a different path. You can follow your heart, and still be in the world, you know. I, for example, am about to go to a peace march."

On Monday night, Joseph has just gone to the tantra Web site to find out what it says about peace when, seemingly out of nowhere, Sharon from marketing plops herself down in his cubicle and stretches out long legs clad in jeans. She peers at him over small black glasses that even he recognizes as very hip and expensive. He tries to block the Web site with his shoulder.

"So what's this tantra thing, Joseph?" she says.

He stares at her, his heart racing. He didn't even think she knew his name.

"Excuse me?"

"Don't worry. I won't tell anybody."

He wonders if she's seen the Web site. But surprisingly, he doesn't feel nervous. "That's too bad," he says. "I think more people should get to know what it is."

"You don't seem like the type of person who would be into it."

"What type of person do I seem like?" He's not flirting. He really wants to know. Have other people noticed a change in him?

Sharon leans back and flicks her black, shiny hair over her shoulder. "I don't know. Why are you here so late every night? Don't you have a girlfriend?"

The thought of being alone with Sharon in the office used to send his imagination soaring. Now he just wishes she would leave. "Why are you here so late?"

"I'm headed home," she says. "Why don't you come over for dinner Saturday night?"

"Sure, that sounds great," he answers, just to get her to go away.

"And then you can tell me more about tantra."

Before Joseph can spit out a response, she's gone. If he didn't think it would set off the smoke alarm, he'd light incense to erase her perfume.

When he gets home that night, he tries to open the golden pipeline, but all he can picture is Sharon's naked body reclining on snow-white sheets. The vision makes him hard, but after he comes, he feels guilty. Every night the rest of the week, Joseph leaves work early to avoid her and goes to the gym for two hours. He's so tired that when he comes home, he falls into bed exhausted, too tired to meditate, much less visit the pipeline. He reasons that he's been opening up his heart every day for the past several months; surely it will stay open if he misses a week or so.

Sharon's apartment is neat and feminine, with large, over-cushioned couches and chairs upholstered in deep plum. She serves him grilled ostrich in a cranberry sauce, potatoes dauphinoise, sautéed spinach and a blood-red burgundy. The food is so rich he can barely taste it. As they sit on the couch after dinner, Joseph realizes that he's slightly drunk. It's a feeling he hasn't had in many months. Sharon wears a low-cut, peach-colored wraparound blouse that shows off her cleavage, and clingy black pants. He is dying to kiss her.

"So," she says. "Tantra."

"How did you know I study tantra?"

"I saw it on your Web site that night. And. . .well, I was in the office the other night, and walked by your cube. You must have been in the bathroom or something."

He pauses. "It's not just about sex."

"Really?" She seems almost disappointed.

"No. It's really a rather esoteric religious practice." He tries to explain to her about kundalini and chakras and sadhana, but her eyes just glaze over. He plunges ahead, afraid to stop. Finally, she interrupts him.

"I just thought tantra was about fucking for hours and hours in wild positions," she says, giggling.

He wants to protest, but he realizes that tantra is the one form of currency he has with her right now. "There are techniques," he says.

"Teach me one." She slides closer to him on the couch.

He stares at her. Three months ago, he would have lunged for her. He would have carried her to the bedroom and slid his hands under that peach-colored blouse. He would have pulled off her pants and slid into her as quickly as he could, plunging again and again into her long-limbed wetness. Now he has a vision of life with her. In an instant he knows what that life would entail, and meditation isn't a part of it. He sees his heart shrinking, and feels a tiny flame of protective anger.

"I have to go," he says, standing up. "Thank you for dinner."

And then something odd happens. Sharon's face crumples, and tears spring into her eyes. "I'm sorry, Joseph. I've offended you."

He sits back down. "No! What's wrong?"

"My mom's really sick," she says. "I just didn't want to be alone tonight."

Joseph takes her hand. "You're not alone. You can talk to me as long as you want. But," he says softly, "I think that should be all."

"I think so, too." She looks up at him, the sophistication and confidence momentarily gone. He has a glimpse of the eight-year-old girl beneath, and he feels his heart expand in his chest.

It's almost four A.M. when Joseph finally gets home. He goes to his bedroom and lies down, staring out at the city. His face is a ghostly reflection in the window. He closes his eyes and sees the golden pipeline, shut down and neglected. He sees it full of sludge and rocks.

He reaches for the phone. He'll just leave a message for Sharon to let her know he's thinking of her and to make sure she's okay. Then he catches himself. *You jerk*, he says to himself affectionately. *You just want to make yourself look good*. He sets the handset back in its cradle. He'll call her when he's clear-headed.

Joseph slips out of his shirt and shorts and lies on his bed. Breathing deeply, he slides his hand down over his stomach. He caresses himself until his penis stirs and hardens. He moves his hand faster and faster. With his other hand, he touches the middle of his chest and rubs it. He imagines pure, hot water flowing through the pipeline between his heart and his hardness, clearing out the debris he'd let accumulate there. Then he imagines the flow of gold starting: first a trickle, then a stream, then an unstoppable torrent circulating the liquid gold in endless circles. He feels the pleasure until he can stand it no longer. Then he lets go, his orgasm pushing out every thought. Afterwards, he dozes, and when he wakes four hours later, he feels as though he's just taken a swim in a cold mountain stream.

The next day, Joseph goes to the café, half hoping that he'll run into Brenda, the nun, again. He sits at a table in the back corner and takes out his book. *Looks like my date today is Pema Chödrön,* he thinks. But only a few minutes have passed before he feels as though someone is watching him. He looks up to see a pretty blonde woman at the next table staring at him over the monitor of her laptop computer. She quickly looks away, then back.

"I'm sorry to stare," she says. "But someone just gave me that book. I'd never heard of it, and all of a sudden, I see it twice in two days. It must be a sign."

"It's the second time I've read it," he says. "I don't think I was paying attention the first time."

She pauses. "I know how that is. I'm Kate, by the way."

"I'm Joseph," he says, and without another thought, adds, "Why don't you join me?"

"I don't usually strike up conversations with strangers," she tells him as she sits down. "But you seem like a really nice person."

Joseph closes his book. He thinks about how her hair looks like the color of molten gold, and smiles.

TANTRIC EXPERIENCE

Open Your Heart with Ecstasy

IF ONLY ALL SPIRITUAL DISCIPLINES WERE AS EASY AND EFFECTIVE as opening your heart through erotic ecstasy! We are all looking for love, but so often in the wrong place. But where is the right place? Not outside, but inside, in your own heart.

Here is a fantastic technique that uses the power of the sexual orgasm to open your heart chakra and deepen your connection to the universal love that lives within it.

This Love Climax technique is fun! In my experience, many meditation techniques are absolutely boring. Not this one! In its essence, tantra is very simple. Once you understand this, then much of the confusion that may surround tantra for you will be cleared up immediately. If you can add 2 + 4, then you can understand the heart of tantra. The tantra of India is a complicated collection of techniques. Only some of it is compatible with our western lifestyles. For example, you could start meditating in graveyards and having sex only at the full moon. If it is your destiny to do these things, then you will, of course. But chances are it is not.

Tantra = 2 + 4. What does this mean? Unify the sex center, the second chakra, with the love center, the fourth chakra. Then you have done tantra. If you accomplish this much, then you have done a very great thing with your life.

To awaken such living love in your body, heart, and mind is a surefire recipe for personal fulfillment. Self-love is the reliable basis for happiness.

In numerology, the number six represents relationships and Venus, the planet of romantic love. Deeply romantic love blends love and sex in a way that maximizes the potential of both: 2 + 4 = 6.

Furthermore, 2 x 4 = 8. This number eight represents the cosmic chakra above the crown chakra at the top of the head. This eighth chakra represents the fully arisen kundalini.

The ultimate romance, according to tantra, is the union of Shiva and Shakti. When that cosmic romance fully blossoms, it is displayed at the eighth chakra, which is universal, not personal. This ultimate experience or state of consciousness is not within your control to create. At best, you can surrender to the Higher Power, to the Universal Love, and ask it to take you there.

Let's first learn the Love Climax technique solo. After a little practice, it will be easy to see how to do it with a partner. As you pleasure yourself, bring your excitement right up to the edge of the climax, but don't go over. The key is to stay comfortable, yet get as close as you can.

Think of standing next to a bonfire at a beach party. You want to feel the heat, but you don't want to get burned! You want to be Orange or close, but not Red and in the fire.

Some students make this stressful. It is meant to be easy and relaxed. If you are straining and struggling, pushing and agonizing trying to stay on the edge, then you are too close. Back off some. As you practice, you are exploring and learning about this high arousal zone. Eventually, it will become effortless to stay there when you want to.

Approach and stay in the high arousal zone at least three times during your Love Climax session. If you can, just hang out, just be, float, flow, melt in that zone. When you feel ready, quickly move your attention up to your heart center in the middle of your chest.

Think of a connection or tube, some kind of energy pipeline, that links the second chakra and the fourth chakra. It's already there, so you don't have to create it. The road has already been built. Now you are going to consciously ride on that energy pathway.

Take your hand and trace the pathway right up the front of your body. There is a natural nerve connection between your genitals and the heart chakra. Can you feel it? You can imagine this tube and make it out of gold or white light, if you like. If you are very visual, that may help you. But you don't have to. It is enough just to know it's there.

While you are still in you high arousal zone, go up to the heart and mentally, inwardly, touch it. If you like, physically touch the center of your chest between your nipples with your free hand. Touch it and feel it for a moment. Do this three times.

You want to keep your attention in the second chakra, in the high arousal zone. So just say "Hi!" and then slide back down to the genitals and to the hot love lava percolating there. The Love Climax technique uses the explosive energy of the sexual orgasm to open the heart chakra. Just putting your mental attention there isn't enough. The extra energy, the concentrated burst of life force from the orgasm, has the power to open your heart more than ever before.

You have brought the energy up to the heart three times, gently tapping there and saying hello. Now, as you go over into the full-blown climax, move your free hand to your chest. Press the palm against your chest and rub there as you climax.

It may help to roll your eyes up and lean your head back. You can visualize light shooting up from your second chakra, from your genitals, to your heart. You can repeat the word "Love! Love! Love!" (or "God!" or a mantra or whatever words work best for you).

Encourage the feeling of swooning, of surrendering and melting and totally letting-go. This is not something you are able to accomplish through effort. It is just the opposite: the more you let go and let the erotic energy flow, glow, and grow, the more you will discover that its natural direction is up—to feed and nourish the heart.

Allow yourself plenty of time to come back. Be prepared to float for five or ten minutes in the afterglow that may follow. This is an important time of integration, where the sex and love centers of your being deepen their intrinsic connections and unify their forces in order to help and heal your life.

First of all, you can secretly do the Love Climax when you make love to your partner. It really is okay. When you make love, bring the energy up to the heart, just as you did when you were self-loving.

You may be fortunate enough to have a partner who wants to do it with you. If so, then the right way to go about this is for each of you to have your own Love Climax sessions on your own. Then you will bring the experience and knowledge from those private self-love sessions to your lovemaking.

What if you don't have a partner right now? Then do the Love Climax and imagine what it would be like to be with a loving partner. Or let your climax energy expand out in a gigantic love explosion from your heart that reaches out to embrace the world with love. This is sex and love magic at its finest.

In the story, Joseph awakens his inner warmth, leaving behind the chill of lackluster loneliness. He discovers that love is about sharing inner treasure, not conquering external appearances. He embarks on a beautiful new journey of falling in love with himself. The organic magnetism that naturally emerges out of that self-love begins to attract people to him. A life of abundance awaits him.

TANTRIC TALE

Lotus Touch

YOU ARE WAITING FOR ME IN A SMALL ADOBE HOUSE AT the end of a grove of eucalyptus trees. I arrive just as the sun abandons the sky, but inside your bedroom, you have just lit twenty candles. They smell like orange blossoms. In the distance, I hear the ocean. You lead me to the bed, and your hazel eyes watch my reaction to the spread you've laid out for me. Honeydew melon. Valencia oranges. Ice water in a cobalt-blue vase. A beaker-shaped decanter of red wine. Tiny chocolate truffles, the size of pebbles, dusted with cocoa powder.

Oh Julia, I say. *You were listening.*

Of course I was listening. Now, don't move. Don't do a thing. Let me give something to you for once.

You reach for me. I stand as motionless as a mannequin as you remove my sandals and unzip my skirt, as you unbutton the mother-of-pearl buttons of my blouse. Your lips trace the curves of my neck. You unhook my bra, then lower your mouth to gently kiss my right nipple, then my left. They harden under the touch of your tongue.

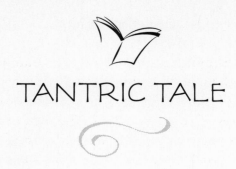

Sorry, you say. *I just had to say hello.*

I want to see you, too.

You smile and pull your dress over your head. I'm glad you're not wearing anything underneath, because it gives me a chance to enjoy the sight of your long dark hair curling over your heavy breasts. The curves of your round hips. The sight of the dark patch of hair between your legs. I rub my body against you so that our hard nipples touch. I can't resist the soft pillows of your full lips. For a moment, our tongues intertwine. Then you pull away, almost roughly.

No touching, you say. *This is your night, remember?*

You lead me to the milk-white sheets of your bed. I lie down so you can pull my panties over my hips. You throw them to the other side of the room with a flourish that makes us both giggle.

What would you like, my love? you whisper.

You know.

Tell me again.

I do.

You roll me onto my stomach, and you begin to touch me. You trace your fingers over my hair, my shoulders, my back, your strokes becoming deeper over my buttocks and thighs. You stroke me all the way down to the tips of my toes, back up, and then down again. But this time, as you come to the tops of my thighs, you slip your fingers to the warm wetness between my legs. I arch against your touch. The tips of your fingers brush that delicate nub that's now hard and aching to be touched; I moan into the pillow. I want you to press harder, but not quite yet. You slide your fingers back up the wetness and then higher, where you pause for a moment.

I feel like I could come right now.

But you pull your hand away and resume your light stroke on my back. It feels as though you're hardly touching me, yet my skin tingles under your touch, as though your hand is pulsing with electricity. Something is happening.

My God, you whisper. *Can you feel that?*

Yes.

Close your eyes.

You roll me over onto my back. Your fingertips trace me, draw me, bring me into being. With my eyes closed, I'm not even sure that you're touching me, but I know exactly where your fingers are at every moment.

Let yourself go, you whisper.

I tremble as you draw spirals on my stomach and hips. You stroke the front of my thighs, and then, easing yourself onto your left side, you lie so close to me I can sense the vibrations of your skin. You slip your fingers between my legs. I am so wet that your middle finger slips off my clitoris for a moment before returning and beginning that quick up-and-down motion I've shown you. I take deep breaths to slow my excitement.

You slide your left hand under me and wet your fingers on my slickness. Then you slide a finger inside and hold it there, so I can feel it as you rub me. Slowly, you begin to move the finger inside me, but not so fast that it distracts me from the pleasure radiating out from my swollen folds. You put another finger at my other, secret entrance. I race up the hill to orgasm, but you pull back just in time. I can sense your eyes on my face, watching me, gauging my pleasure.

Again and again you take me to the edge, until I forget where or who I am. I feel as though I'm merging with the night sky and the ocean in the distance. My hips buck against your hand; my legs stiffen against the bed. Finally, I can take no more.

Now, I cry. *Oh God, now.*

You plunge your fingers in and out of me, and then I'm coming, and coming, and coming, my head crashing into the soft down of your pillows. For an instant, I feel like I am floating on a cushion of light.

And then I'm back.

I am helpless. You feed me cubes of honeydew from fingers that are still wet. They scent the fruit with my own musky perfume. You hold a glass of wine to my lips, and as the liquid slides over my tongue, I taste blackberries and coffee and deep, rich earth. A breeze ruffles your white curtains and brings the eucalyptus trees into the room, the room that pulsates with our love.

Tomorrow, it will be your turn.

But now you help me to my feet, wrap a cotton robe around me, and lead me down to the beach, where waves of salt water lap against my toes and bring me back to myself, and to you.

TANTRIC EXPERIENCE

Share Sexual Rapture Now

PARTNER SEX IS NOT THE ONLY WAY TO HAVE GREAT SEX. Some of my best sexual experiences have been by myself. That's not because I'm a lousy lover. Nor have my lovers been bad in bed. The key is that I know what I want, how I want it, when I want it, and at what intensity—moment to moment to moment. That is the key to SRI, too.

SRI is an acronym for "Sexual Rapture Intensive." SRI is also a mantra pronounced "Shree." This is a sacred sound of the Goddess of Love, Beauty, and Abundance, of the energy called Aphrodite or Venus. If you repeat "Shree" or "Shreem" silently or out loud while being sexually pleasured, it will make you more sensitive to the subtle flows of energy in your body and increase your bliss. Like the OM, it expresses the eternal love song of the universe.

SRI enables you to achieve altered states of bliss, rapture, and joy like the high states of classic meditation while you deepen your love connection through beautiful sexual bonding. With the help of SRI, you learn how to give your partner heavenly sexual pleasure. They will cry tears of ecstasy and of joy even as they gain insights into love, life, and the spiritual self.

Because SRI involves long periods of manual stimulation, you will need a good lubricant and plenty of it. In the Red Hot Resources section, I mention some excellent products. If you're on a limited budget, try almond oil. Experiment until you find a lubricant that feels wonderful on your skin and you both love to use. Just remember that if you use an oil-based lubricant, and then have intercourse with a condom, that condom will be compromised. It you think you will be using a condom, use water-based lubricants only. Or have a shower first to wash off the oil-based product.

Put the lubricant in a big squeeze bottle, perhaps one from a massage products store. That way you can squirt it as needed without breaking your rhythm. Have clean towels, music CDs, snacks, and spring water on hand.

SRI is a manual stimulation approach. Most people can keep up a steady stimulation using their hand(s) for twenty minutes or more. You will need to maintain a consistent rhythm the whole time. Prolonged genital stimulation results in a "steady state" of ecstasy that feels, more or less, like one long orgasm. Sometimes, SRI takes the Receiver into mystical, illuminated states.

Once your partner has reached a peak level like this and had some good climaxes—in the case of the male, without ejaculation—take a five-minute break. After you resume stimulation, your partner will quickly return to their peak level.

SRI is not a substitute for your regular lovemaking. In fact, you will appreciate intercourse and oral sex even more. Doing SRI together deepens your ability to feel and enjoy all the forms of sexual pleasure that you share. Echoing the timeless dance of Yin and Yang, one partner is the Giver, the other partner is the Receiver. You may think that the Giver has the hard part. In fact, most people have more difficulty with the role of Receiver.

The Receiver has permission to focus on herself and claim her erotic joy. She is permitted to be selfish and receive pure pleasure with no obligation to give it back. The Receiver is asserting her right to have this pleasure. The Receiver needs to tell the Giver what she wants. The Giver cannot read her mind. If the Receiver isn't sure what to ask for, the Giver goes ahead and starts giving her pleasure.

The Receiver lies on her back on the bed unless another position is preferred.

As pleasure builds for the Receiver, she will probably tune into what she wants most in the moment. Being assertive, she tells her partner "Joe, I don't like the up and down on me so much. Could you try side to side?" Or "Faster, Joe. Go really fast and keep the steady rhythm. I'm so close!"

The Giver may get bored or think their actions are mechanical. The motions are repetitive, but they are giving the Receiver a fantastic experience of pleasure. Not only is this a priceless gift, sooner or later, the Giver gets to receive!

A man at a tantric retreat near Toronto, Canada, complained that he felt like "a human vibrator." I replied, "Why do you think vibrators are so popular?" The group exploded with laughter.

As rapport builds, you may experience a kind of sexual ESP. You are intuitively synchronized, and the need for words is transcended. But do not expect intuitive rapport to tell you all you need to build arousal up to maximum intensity. Use words until they fall away naturally in the ecstasy.

However, the Giver does not rely just on what the Receiver tells him. He watches and listens very closely to the Receiver. With practice, these skills become art. The Giver plays the Receiver's body and makes music with it. When you reach a plateau of high sexual arousal, Giver and Receiver work together to keep the Receiver near the edge. Here, a woman may have multiple orgasms. A man may have multiple orgasms, too, without ejaculation.

Eventually, the Receiver is ready to go over the edge. The Receiver may ask for it. Or you may know the Receiver well enough that you can tell when they are done "peaking" (or "plateau-ing") and are ready to go over their Niagara Falls into a spectacular, body-blasting, mind-dissolving climax.

For some Receivers, there will be a need to cushion the reentry. At first, words may not be possible. Just hold each other. Listen to the music.

SRI builds up a tremendous sexual charge. The orgasm energy is kept in the sex chakra, stirring up the mystical kundalini power and drawing it up from its home in the root chakra and in the earth itself.

Afterwards, eat substantial food. Drink plenty of water. The Receiver may want a soothing shower. You may want to come down by showering together or sharing a hot tub. But if the Receiver is spaced out, a cold shower alone is best. Definitely do *not* get in a car and drive right away, especially if you were the Receiver! Check for any signs of being spaced out before you drive.

Now that you know the basics of SRI, you must actually do the SRI technique. Set aside an hour or two and do it. Go on a tantric weekend retreat and do it. Tantra is about experience. Tantra without experience is tantrum—the drama of frustration.

Write your SRI experiences down in your Red Hot Diary. Just a brief paragraph is enough. Include the date and setting. Later, when you want to review and relive these magnificent peak experiences, you will be delighted that you wrote them down. Your erotic life will keep getting better as you travel this self-educational spiral.

In the story, Julia and her lover explore the wonder of the senses together. They focus wordlessly on the miracle of touch. They melt into the enchanted skies that smile over love's sweet ocean.

Julia and her lover demonstrate exquisite tantric taste for set and setting. In this atmosphere of loving surrender, the deep bliss of immortal tantric truths is released, not only to them, but for the benefit of the world.

TANTRIC TALE

Skintensity

SHE DECIDES THAT TONIGHT WILL BE THE NIGHT SHE teaches him about touch. She decides this in a most unlikely place: a taqueria in the Mission. She decides it as she watches him pour hot sauce onto a carne asada burrito, add a tiny mountain of jalapeños, and wolf it down. His appetites turn her on. He gobbles life. He gobbles her. But does he use all of his senses? After a year with him, she's still not sure. She plays with the tiny diamond stud in her nose.

"Dude, what're you thinking about?" he asks.

As he waits for her answer, he washes down his burrito with the last of his beer, and signals for another one. She ticks off the senses. Taste. Smell. Those are easy. He definitely uses those.

"I'm thinking about what I'm going to do to you later. And don't call me dude."

He grins at her, feline. His eyes dart to her cleavage in her black tank top, and his grin grows wider.

Sight. Hearing. Of course. He's a bike messenger. Those senses have to be well-developed, or he couldn't do his job. She has an image of him pedaling up and down hilly streets, weaving in and out of traffic with a cat's grace. It's the same image she conjures during the day to make her receptionist job less boring. She's jealous of his freedom, of the energy that makes him so good at what he does. Fast. Agile. Instinctual. He's never had an accident. When he rides, he's attuned to everything around him. Why isn't he attuned to her?

Touch. That's it. That's the one he's missing. The most neglected of the senses. She will teach him.

She smiles. He has no idea what she has in mind.

"Don't drink any more," she tells him.

"Okay," he says without hesitation.

She wants to laugh out loud at how completely he trusts her.

They go to a dark basement club and dance until their clothes are soaked with sweat. His energy never flags. Back in her tiny studio, surrounded by her half-finished paintings, he comes to bed aroused. His penis juts out from his lithe body like the prow of a ship. She loves that the idea of her makes him so hard night after night. She just wants it to last. She wants *him* to last.

At least he's not one of those guys who lose interest after the initial conquest, she thinks. Quite the opposite. When it comes to their sex life, it seems to her as though he shifts up a gear every month. But as his lust and his familiarity with her body have grown, the length of their lovemaking has decreased. At the beginning, they'd go for hours. Now, she's lucky if he lasts five minutes. She can't decide whether he's being efficient or just lazy. To his credit, he always turns to her after he's had his own orgasm, and he won't give up until she's come, too. But she's tired of these abbreviated lovemaking sessions. They leave her hungry.

"Lie back," she tells him. He complies. *He thinks he's going to get the best blow job of his life,* she thinks, smiling to herself.

Instead she rolls him onto his stomach.

"Hey," he says, protesting mildly. He's protective of his ass. He has this idea—she doesn't know where it came from, nor does he—that if he leaves it unguarded, she'll pull out her dildo and harness, strap it on, and ravage him. She suspects it's actually his fantasy, but she's not going to push it. Not tonight.

"Relax," she says. She pours some massage oil into the palm of her hand. She touches him lightly in long, feathery strokes.

"A massage? Dude, you're going to make me fall asleep."

"No, I won't. Just be quiet and think about my fingers on you. And don't call me dude."

She keeps her strokes light and fast, as though his body were a canvas that she has to prime. With each stroke of her fingers over his shoulder blades, down the small of his back, over his firm buttocks to his strong thighs and calves, she wipes the canvas clean. She moves back to his shoulders and pulls her fingertips down his triceps, his forearms, his palms, and his fingertips. She imagines she can feel the humming of his nerves. For a moment, she can.

"Wow, babe. My skin is tingling."

"Shhhh. Or I'll stop."

Now she has to dust him. She knows that painters don't do this to their canvases, but it seems right to her. She takes out the feather duster from under the bed and touches it lightly over his skin.

"What's that? That feels cool."

"Shhhhh."

She rolls him onto his back.

"Get on top of me."

"Do I have to gag you to keep you quiet?" She reaches into her drawer and takes out a black silk blindfold. He lets her tie it around his head. Then, she kneels next to him and pours some more massage oil into her palm. Now she strokes the front of his body, imagining that she is no longer a painter but a sculptor, and his skin is made of clay. She touches the place where his pulse beats in his neck and follows the tendons of his neck down to his chest. She frets his nipples lightly and runs her palms over his rib cage. Pausing at the small tattoo of a Celtic knot on his right hip, she sculpts his flat stomach and draws a ring around his penis. *I'll come back to you,* she tells it. She barely touches his balls before moving on to his thighs, his knees, his shins, his feet.

"That tickles," he whispers. "But in a good way." She's surprised to hear that the resistance has disappeared from his voice, replaced by awe. The room's energy shifts, quiets, comes alive. Wherever her fingers touch his body, she imagines sparks.

"Just focus on the sensations." She takes the feather duster and touches the feathers to his stiffness. His hips thrust up—involuntarily, it seems—to meet them.

"Sorry. I couldn't help it."

"That's okay."

She straddles him and sits lightly on his hips. She feels his penis press against the small of her back.

She takes his hands in hers. "Don't try to move them. Let me do it."

Gently, taking a deep breath, she touches his fingers to her chest so that he can feel its smoothness. She moves his fingers over the fullness of her breasts. She pretends his fingers are her own and uses them to touch her nipples, fondling them until they're hard. She traces the curve of her waist, the swelling of her hips, rising up so he can feel the soft roundness of her buttocks.

"I love your ass," he whispers. "God, I love your ass."

Usually, she would make a comment about its size, but now she feels it as he does—her ass is voluptuous, a juicy, olive-skinned honeydew melon. Perfect. Smiling, she moves his hands between her legs and puts his thumb on her clitoris, rubbing it back and forth a few times.

He groans. She can see how hard he is and almost takes pity on him. Almost.

Using his fingers, she rubs herself until she feels like the wetness will drip down on him. Then, slowly, she lowers herself onto his erection. She savors the feeling of it entering her inch by inch until finally, her hips meet his. With his thumb still on her, she continues to rub herself. She puts his other hand back on her breast.

"Oh, God," he moans. He tries to thrust. He reaches for the blindfold.

She grabs his hand and pushes it to the bed. "Don't move."

She tightens herself around him and begins to move up and down on it, slowly at first, then faster. She rocks her pelvis against his finger.

"Slow down, babe. I'm getting really close."

She's surprised. Usually, he wouldn't tell her. She stops, rests.

Now he moves his fingers, and she lets him. He rubs her hard nub and then her nipples, sending waves of pleasure deep into her womb. She feels her lips soften and swell around him. She puts her hands down on either side of him and braces herself.

"Keep going," she whispers.

"You feel so wet. So warm."

"Keep going."

She returns her hands to his chest. She wants to feel his skin. She is nothing but sensations. He seems to sense it, too, and keeps his hands on her as he starts thrusting upwards, gently at first, and then harder. He takes his time. Five minutes. Ten. Finally, it's enough. Her orgasm explodes inside her, and as she starts to come, he takes his hand away from her breasts and clutches her ass, cementing her body against him.

She collapses onto him, her soft breasts against his firm chest. Through her skin, she feels his heart beating. Their breathing returns to normal. She reaches up and removes his blindfold, and he gazes at her as though for the first time. He no longer needs her guiding fingers. He strokes her skin himself.

"I didn't come," he says in wonder. He is still hard inside her. "Sweet."

He reaches for the blindfold, and ties it around her eyes. Now, it can be his turn. He rolls over with her until she's on her back, and balancing on his hands, begins to thrust into her, but slowly. Her hips rock to meet his. She feels every inch of him.

"Go slow," he whispers, and then says the words she's wanted to hear for months. "I want to feel you. I want to feel you for a long time."

TANTRIC EXPERIENCE

Make Love Blindfolded

BE HERE NOW. HOW?

Here is a powerful, playful way to leap into the here and now! Blindfold the eyes, and instantly your other senses rush forward to fill up your experience. Try it right now. Close your eyes for ten seconds. Go ahead.

Good. Closing your eyes is relaxing. Some people meditate with their eyes closed. The eyes place the greatest demand on the brain's resources—68 percent, according to one expert. Just imagine what kind of party your other senses can have when two-thirds of your brain's capacity is suddenly set free.

Let's try it again, only this time I would like you to actively explore your experience by visiting each sense and being with it for a few moments. With your eyes closed, go to your eardrums and *listen*. Then go to your skin and your sense of touch and *feel*. Go to your nostrils and *smell*. Then go to your tongue and *taste*.

The order in which you do this doesn't really matter. Follow the order that is natural for you. Your purpose is simply to visit all the senses.

Finally, go to your eyes and feel the muscles behind them. These muscles anchor your eyes in your brain. They tend to get rigid. Relax those muscles. Let the eyeballs go soft, like jelly. You may feel a wave of relief and relaxation as the muscles and eyeballs soften. Experience your eyes as physical soft tissue. Sense the weight and substance of them. Feel the space within and around each eye.

Smile. Did you enjoy this inner journey?

Actively exploring each sense makes closing your eyes more rewarding. Entering into the spaciousness of each sense deepens meditation. Blindfolds take this journey of self-discovery up a notch. Sensual and elegant, silk is the perfect fabric choice. I prefer red silk because it seems sexy to me, but you may prefer black. Elegant facemasks are sold in red and black, too.

When you do this with a partner, close your eyes at the same time and do the sense exploration. Then you choose who is blindfolded and the fun begins.

Classic "tricks" include stroking your blindfolded partner with a feather, feeding them chocolate-coated strawberries and other sensual foods, and dripping ice water from a melting ice cube on their skin. I would like to show you how to take this fun blindfold game to a deeper level.

Take your blindfolded partner by the hand for a walk around your home. Have them touch, taste, smell, and listen to things in your home. A few minutes of this will do. If your partner is really enjoying this exploration, then let them continue, of course. Now lead them back to the bed and give them a brief massage using thick, rich oil like jojoba or almond. When you are done giving them the massage, tell them you are going to kiss them.

However, this is a trick! Don't kiss them. Wait until they say something like "Where's my kiss?"

"It's coming," you say. Then kiss them somewhere other than their lips. After a few kisses on different parts of their body, kiss them on the lips very lightly, then lift away. Kiss them again and again, with a pause in between. Linger longer each time until, finally, you lay a long, wet one on them.

It is said that the most important—or the biggest—sex organ lies between the ears. It is your brain. That's why this little love game works.

Now tell them, "I would like to make love to you." Wait for their response. If they are open to trying that with the blindfold on, let them totally receive and be as passive as they like. They are in a state of meditation. Of course, do not force this experience on them.

I have asked groups "What was the most beautiful erotic experience of your life?" One answer I have heard repeatedly over the years from both men and women is "Being made love to while blindfolded."

How will you know if making love blindfolded is right for you? You will just have to try it and see!

In the story, a young painter blindfolds her bike messenger boyfriend and takes him for the ride of his life. She paints his body with her fingers, showing him a new vision of lovemaking. Words, as likely to divide as they are to conquer, are utterly transcended. The love, when spoken, is from the heart. Dropping from the mind, diving into the stream of natural being that is the body, they discover in the language of the skin the living message of love.

TANTRIC TALE

Mudra

On the third night of their honeymoon in Bali, Roxanna wakes from a dream sweating and horny. Next to her, François sleeps soundly, exhausted from a day of diving. Roxanna listens to the waves rolling against the beach. A slight breeze moves palm fronds outside their window, casting shadows on the wall. The door to their balcony stands ajar. All is calm, peace. Why does she feel so restless, as if a thunderstorm were on the horizon? The sheets stick to her like wet ropes. She reaches between her legs and finds that she is swollen and moist.

The dream comes back to her. She is wandering through the Pasar Ubud marketplace, but none of the wares appeal to her. She walks past the Pura Dalem Agung, the Temple of the Dead, to the Monkey Forest Sanctuary. Long-tailed macaques stop their chattering to watch her silently. She comes to a clearing and sits on the ground. She waits: for what, she isn't sure.

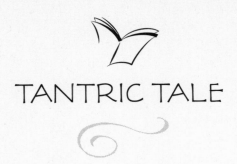

A young, red-skinned woman emerges from the other side of the clearing. Dark-haired, dark-eyed, she is dressed in red silk, and on her head sits a crown of five skulls. Under her left arm is a shaft of some sort. She brims with youth and vitality; she glows around the edges as though there were a halo of fire behind her. In her dream mind, Roxanna understands that this woman is a goddess and wants to shield her eyes. But she can't move her head: The woman holds Roxanna in the intensity of her gaze. Roxanna realizes that the goddess has a third eye in the center of her forehead, but this fact does not frighten the dreaming Roxanna; in fact, it calms her.

The woman begins to move in a graceful, sinuous dance that seems, improbably, both spontaneous and ritualized. Her bejeweled hands twist in the air. The woman's robes begin to open as if an invisible lover were undressing her, and as they fall to the ground, Roxanna marvels at the smooth olive skin and flowing curves of the woman's body, her full breasts with their pointed nipples, her round hips and belly, her heavy legs, the lush patch of dark pubic hair between her legs. A necklace of human skulls swings from her neck. In her left hand, she holds a golden skullcap. She tips the bowl toward Roxanna, who sees that it is filled with blood. Roxanna understands that it is menstrual blood, but she is still not afraid.

The woman smiles at Roxanna. Her dance quickens and grows more vigorous; her feet whirl around the forest floor. The only sound is the clacking of her necklace of skulls against the bone ornaments that encircle her body. Suddenly she stops on her left toes, her body suspended in the air. The thumb and index finger of her right hand pinch her left nipple. With the index and fourth finger of her left hand, the woman has parted the swollen lips between her legs, and Roxanna sees, with a shock of desire, that her third finger rubs the hard nub between the folds.

And that was when Roxanna woke up.

She nudges François until his eyes open.

"You must touch me," she whispers. "I saw a goddess."

"You're dreaming, my love," he mumbles, reluctant to leave his own dream world.

But when he sees how her long, black, curly hair falls around her face and pools on the pillow, and how her brown-black eyes shimmer, and how the bed sheets curl around her legs, he wakes fully. He reaches for her, and his mouth seeks the place where her neck meets her shoulder.

"Touch me like this," she says, and shows him, arranging her hands in the mudra of the goddess.

He pushes the sheets off her body. Once she is completely naked, he begins to caress her in the usual way, the way that has always worked for her. But this time, she stops him.

"No," she says. "Like this." And again she shows him.

He takes one of her nipples between his fingers, and with his other hand, seeks the soft folds between her legs. He draws in his breath when he feels how wet she is. His finger searches through the dense hair for the soft nub. Carefully, firmly, he starts to rub it as he rolls her nipple between his fingers. He bends his head to her other nipple and begins to suck it.

Roxanna feels as though someone has attached her to a live electrical current that runs directly from her sex to her nipple. She arches and groans, and François is wise enough to keep his hands on her as he rubs harder. She comes faster than she ever has before, with an orgasm that pulses through her body like the shock waves of an underwater earthquake. As she comes, everything around her dissolves—the room, the bed, the hotel, even François. She thrashes in the bed.

Afterwards, François kisses and holds her, and as she falls asleep, she sees, once again, the mysterious smile of the goddess, and her hands, twisting like vines.

TANTRIC EXPERIENCE

Nipple Attunement

SOME WOMEN ARE ABLE TO EXPERIENCE ORGASM FROM breast and nipple stimulation alone, proving that the nipples and genitals are intimately linked or hard-wired. More importantly, the nipples are one of the links in an invisible electrical ecstasy circuit that connects genitals, nipples, mouth, and brain.

Tantric theory asserts that the highest ecstasy resides in the chakras in the head. Fortunately, you don't have to try to jump from the genitals straight up to the crown. By shifting the attention gradually upwards, you pull the sexual energy with it. As energy centers connect, ecstasy increases and emotions open. The body lights up with energy. The result is whole-body arousal and climax, even mystical experiences.

In *Open Your Heart with Ecstasy,* I helped you raise your sensations of sexual arousal to your heart. Here I want to show you how to get in touch with the entire energy circuit in the front of the body. The energy circuit in the back of the body is, of course, the spine.

The heart is located midway between the genitals and the mouth. The heart is the next step on your feeling journey to the "no-mind" bliss of the crown.

You have probably read about your body's energy centers. Here is a tantric meditation guaranteed to make you feel the inner electrical connection between the centers associated with the genitals, nipples, tongue, and crown.

Sit or lie down with your legs wide open. If you are sitting, no crossed legs or ankles, please. Put your feet flat on the floor.

Imagine that you are being genitally pleasured. Naturally, you can do this by stimulating yourself and stopping, but only a little wave or tickle of good feeling in the genitals is needed. Or you can touch or hold your genitals, just maintaining a steady sensation there.

Reach across your chest and grasp your left nipple with your right hand. Squeeze. Note the response. Let go. Now grasp your right nipple with your left hand. Squeeze. Note the response. Let go. Feel the reverberations of sensation.

Which nipple is more sensitive?

Return to the more sensitive nipple. Squeeze fairly hard—hard enough that it keeps your attention, but not so hard that you resist it. The pressure on your nipple should feel slightly painful, yet still be pleasurable. One way to find this level is to squeeze harder and harder until it is too much, then back down from that intensity a notch or two.

Again imagining that your genitals are receiving pleasurable stimulation (in whatever way *you* would like), close your eyes and feel the connection between your nipple and your sex. Notice how introducing the nipple sensation creates a resonant field between them. Genital stimulation by itself or nipple stimulation by itself is not the same as both at the same time. Let go of one or the other, and you will sense this. If you cannot feel the dance of energy between them, chances are you need to intensify your nipple play.

Enjoy that fusion for a minute. Continuing to feel this connected arousal of genitals and nipple, notice what is taking place at your mouth. In your relaxing and opening to the genital and chest pleasures, it may have opened instinctively.

If it is not open, open it wide. Now stick your tongue out. Really stick it out! Stick it out so that it is firm and strong and horizontal, not resting on your lips, like it suddenly has a life of its own.

Make a statement with your tongue—I am free! I am claiming my ecstasy! Now when you look at a traditional statue of the Hindu goddess Kali, and see her sticking out her red tongue, you will understand her unusual gesture in a new way.

Move your jaw and loosen it up. Once your jaw is comfortable, continue breathing with your tongue out. On the surface of your tongue, you will feel how the air is cooler as it comes in over your tongue, warmer as it goes out.

Your eyes are closed. You are imagining pleasurable genital stimulation. You have one hand gently (or not so gently) squeezing the opposite nipple. Your tongue is sticking out. Continue for one minute. Relax and let go of tension in the face, in the shoulders, in the chest and belly.

Can you feel your body unifying itself into an energized whole?

Now for the finishing touch. With your free hand, get a good grip on your hair and pull it up. Pull hard so that it hurts a little. Use the same approach you used to arrive at the right nipple pressure—enough but not too much. (If you are bald, then pat the back of your head rapidly).

Don't worry about how you look. Just explore the opening that is taking place from these strong sensations. There are no words to describe what you may discover by doing this. It may take you into the primal "no-mind" state.

Try it again, but leave an element out. For example, don't squeeze the nipple. It will not be the same. Or keep the mouth closed. Or let go of your hair. You will sense a difference.

Instead of imagining genital stimulation, you can tighten your anal muscles, pulling up and in. It may also help to be attentive to the soles of your feet, especially if you are sitting down. Then you will feel the energy going from your feet to the top of your head.

Now let's turn this tantric meditation into a tantric sexual peak experience. For the nipple stimulation, use wooden clothespins. They are gentler than the plastic variety. In a store, you can discreetly test the pressure on the webbed area of your hand. At home, you can test them on your own nipples until you find one that has just the right pressure.

Don't leave the pins on for more than twenty minutes. Depending on your tolerance, five minutes is fine. If you can't handle more than thirty seconds or so, then that particular clothespin is too tight for you. Part of your reward is the sensitivity that follows after the pin is gently lifted off the nipple. Depending on the intensity of stimulation, this can last for hours. Frequent nipple play awakens permanent nipple sensitivity in both men and women.

Attach a wooden clothespin to each nipple. Remember, you have already tested these pins and they are just right. Now begin pleasuring yourself. If your partner is willing to lend a hand, so much the better!

Relax, let go, and feel the connection between your genitals and your nipples. This is very important—breathe! If you are holding your breath, notice this and let the breath go. Breathe a little more deeply and rhythmically than you usually do. The key is to keep the breath full and rhythmic. It does not have to be dramatic.

Now add Kali's hard, red-hot tongue. Stick your tongue out proudly. Now breathe through your mouth, feeling the air moving in and out over your tongue. If you like, make a panting sound.

Now the piéce de rèsistance! Grab your hair and yank hard! As you pull up firmly on your hair, roll your eyes up. Not so far backwards that you feel a strain on them, but enough to feel a slight swooning effect. It may help to lean back. If you are on a chair, be sure it is stable. Do *not* try this on a chair with rollers, such as the kind found in offices!

Surrender. Surrender to your own circuitry. Surrender to your own deep self. Surrender to your natural, free, uninhibited state, beyond any boundaries or limitations. Surrender to this whole-body pure aliveness feeling.

You may feel a strong, even electrical connection, between your nipples and your clitoris or penis. This is good, but the tantric level is to taste and embrace the whole-body unbounded state without blocks or thinking.

I guarantee that this technique will get you in touch with your wild tantric self. You may even have an experience of ego loss or return to some primal surrendered state beyond words or names, beyond the mind. It is as powerful as it is simple, for it is physically opening and connecting all the centers that were open and connected in you as a baby, when you were still living in a natural state of whole-body ecstasy.

Anytime you want to expand energy up and through your body during lovemaking or self-pleasuring, stimulate the nipples, stick out the tongue, and pull on the hair. These tricks automatically move the energy through the body. Ask your partner to pull on your hair and see what happens!

For men, it will help them delay ejaculation as well as intensify orgasms. For women, it may open new doors of sensation as well as make the earth move like never before.

In the story, Roxanna dreams of a goddess figure who resembles Kali, the spiritual mistress of total sexual ecstasy and freedom. In that dream, this goddess of her inner guidance shows her the link between her nipples and her clitoris. With the help of her partner, François, she is able to realize this connection and, at least for a moment, dissolve into the primal unity that is the secret truth of all sexual activities, of life and love itself.

5

CHAPTER FIVE

Tantric Seeing

TANTRIC TALE

I Am the Light

On a hot afternoon in late August, Carrie sits in a large wood-beamed room of a retreat center in New Mexico, waiting for her massage therapist. Through the large picture window, she watches the setting sun redden the desert mountains and then turn them the color of amethysts. She tries to meditate on them—then on a cactus, and when that doesn't work, on a rock—but try as she might, she can't detach from her feeling of anticipation. She wishes that Michael were here with her. She hasn't seen her husband since morning, when he left their room with a kiss and a promise that he'd see her later that evening.

He's made her many promises lately. The first was when he convinced her to come to this place. Holding her hands tightly across their tiny kitchen table, he'd promised her that this retreat would help them take their relationship to another level. Though they have been practicing yoga and meditation for years, she was skeptical—another one of Michael's spiritual "experiments"—but when she saw photographs of the mountains in the four-color brochure, she agreed to come without a moment's hesitation.

Then, this morning, Michael made his second promise: that the massage she's about to have will be different than anything she's ever experienced. She pinned him on the bed and tried to tickle the secret out of him; when that didn't work, she tried covering his dimpled checks with kisses. But he would only say he wanted it to be a surprise.

Have an open heart, she says to herself, repeating the refrain she's heard at the beginning of every meditation since they arrived. *Have an open mind.*

"Carrie?"

She looks up and stops herself from gasping. Standing in front of her is one of the most handsome men she's ever seen. His loose white T-shirt does nothing to hide his muscled upper body and biceps. His black hair is pulled neatly back into a ponytail; his skin is the color of toast; and when he smiles, his straight, white teeth gleam. *He could be Native American,* she thinks. Or he could be from India. She can't tell his age, either. He could be twenty-five; he could be forty-five.

He speaks in a voice like honey. "I'm Rick. I'm your therapist this evening."

When he reaches out his hand to shake hers, she instantly relaxes. Something about him makes her feel utterly safe. *The Dalai Lama's presence in Mr. Universe's body,* she thinks to herself, and smiles as she follows him, puppy-like, to the treatment room. A group of scented candles burn in one corner, filling the room with the smell of sandalwood and jasmine. In the other corner, water trickles over the pebbles in a small fountain. On one wall, she notices a chart showing the location of the chakras; on the opposite wall is a framed print depicting a scene from the Kama Sutra. *The Kama Sutra?* she thinks. She's never seen that in a massage room.

But she doesn't have time to think about it: The next thing she notices is that Michael, all six feet of him, is standing in one corner of the room. She wants to reach out and run her fingers through his tousled dark blond hair. He beams at her, the dimples in his cheeks deepening.

"Hi, honey," he says. "Surprise!"

"What are you doing here, sweetheart?"

"I'm learning to give you something new," he answers.

She steals a glance at Rick. She once joked with Michael about her fantasy of getting a sensual massage from two men at once. Is that what this is? And if it is, is she ready for it? She feels a wave of nervousness. But Rick smiles gently and puts his hand on her shoulder.

"I'm going to walk Michael through the beginning of the massage, but he will complete it," he says. "And at one point, I'll leave the room. Meanwhile, all you have to do is relax. Tonight is your night to receive."

He turns his back as she slips out of her robe and under the sheet on the table. She takes one last look at Michael before putting her head on the face cradle.

"Carrie, are you ready to take your bodywork to another level?" asks Rick. His voice floats somewhere above her right shoulder.

"Yes."

"First, I'm going to remove the sheet. Is that okay with you?"

She's never been completely naked during a massage before, but she trusts him. "Sure."

He folds back the sheet, then removes it. The warm air of the room caresses her bottom. She sighs and imagines herself on a beach, the sun on her skin.

"Michael," Rick says. "Put one of your hands here—" she feels Rick's hand touch her between her shoulder blades—"and the other here." He rests his hand on the small of her back. He removes his hands, and she feels Michael's.

Michael begins to rock her. The room fills with silence, thick as incense. A lump rises in her throat, catching her off-guard; she breathes deeply and reminds herself that she is safe.

"Now try this," Rick says. He kneads Carrie's back as though he is a baker subduing a dense ball of dough. Long flowing strokes become deep circular ones. Then she feels Michael's hands do the same thing. Rick rakes his fingers down her back, over her butt and down her thighs. His hands glide over the base of her spine and mould her buttocks. Each stroke is followed by Michael's, who finds and dislodges the tension hiding in her body, like smooth, hidden pebbles lodged in the long, lean rivers of her muscles.

Carrie forgets where she is. She almost forgets *who* she is. She feels like she's floating, but soon she feels something else, too.

Aroused.

She knows that if Michael were to slip his hands between the soft folds of her lower lips, his fingers would come away wet. In fact, she wishes that Rick would leave the room so that she could pull Michael onto her.

"Carrie, could you turn over, please?" Rick says.

She flips over without protest, but she keeps her eyes closed. She knows, somehow, that what is happening is not about sex. It is preparing her for something. Standing behind her head, Rick slips his hands under her shoulders, hooking his fingers deep under her shoulder blades, and almost lifts her off the table as he slides his hands up to her neck, over her shoulders and down over her chest, again and again. Then Michael takes over. His strokes move out from her breastbone to her armpits until she feels her chest expand.

"Where did you learn to do that?" Carrie asks.

"Rick is an amazing teacher. Keep breathing, love. Smooth, deep breaths."

"Michael, you can take it from here," Rick says softly.

Michael spreads oil over her belly and thighs. He puts one hand below her rib cage; the other, below her navel. Carrie tenses—she's always felt strange about having her stomach touched—but Michael waits until she feels the tightness in her belly relax, then begins sliding his hands in large, circular strokes around Carrie's abdomen. He decreases the circles, then expands them outwards once again. Carrie feels her breathing deepen. Finally, he slows, then stops, leaving one hand on her belly.

Rick places a gentle hand on Carrie's forehead. "Carrie, I'm going to leave you in Michael's capable hands," he whispers.

As soon as she hears the door close, she feels Michael's lips meet hers, parting them with his tongue.

"I want you," Carrie says. She takes his hand and touches his fingers to her wetness.

"Not yet," he replies. "Remember, tonight, you're receiving." She opens her eyes to see him take a small brown bottle from a shelf.

"That's a nice place to keep the lube," she says.

He smiles. "It's not lube. It's clove oil. I'm going to dab some on your forehead."

"Is *that* the surprise?" She can't tell whether she's relieved or disappointed.

"In a way. It's a tool to achieve the surprise. You're just going to have to trust me."

"I already do." The act of talking seems to require superhuman effort.

Michael touches his finger to Carrie's forehead like a benediction. The clove oil stings slightly and gives off a sweet, strangely rich fragrance. An image—a tiny mountain of brown cane sugar, aflame—flashes in her mind. As the mountain burns, it turns a deep indigo blue.

"Keep your eyes closed, honey," Michael says softly.

He moves his mouth down her body. He kisses her breasts, sucks briefly on her nipples, and touches his lips to her belly. He teases her navel with his tongue, then moves around the end of the massage table and kisses the soles of her feet. Her ankles. Her thighs. He gently kisses the soft, furry mound between her legs. When he speaks, his voice is low, husky. She knows this means he is aroused, too.

"When you're ready, roll your eyes up and look at the place where the clove oil is touching your skin. Look at it from the inside. That's where your mind's eye is. Your third eye. That's where the visions come from."

"Visions?"

He nuzzles her pubic hair. She thinks that if he doesn't begin licking her soon, she'll explode. "You're a visual person, my love," he murmurs against her thigh. "You even talk about your orgasms visually. This will help you focus. When you come, roll your eyes up and keep them focused on the clove oil."

He kisses her outer lips, and then licks the inner ones, his tongue strong and insistent. He teases her clitoris with his tongue, then starts licking it, flicking it faster and faster until it's hard as a river stone. Soon, she feels the strumming of nerves deep within her. Her fingers clench the sheet covering the massage table.

Michael slides a finger into her, holding it there so she can clench around it. Still, his tongue doesn't let up, and involuntarily, her hips begin to rock. He begins moving his finger in and out of her, slowly. She imagines him inside her, and another wave of excitement flashes through her like the rhythm of thunder beyond the mountains.

"I'm getting close," she whispers.

He lifts his head momentarily. "Keep focusing on the oil," he says. He bends his head to her once again and redoubles his efforts.

She rolls her eyes up to meet the clove oil and locks them. The orgasm comes upon her like a flash flood, and suddenly, she is no longer in the room. She is standing on top of a mountain—she knows intuitively that it is one of the mountains at which she gazed earlier—but the desert below has disappeared under an ocean, the waves roiling below lightning bolts and claps of thunder. Strange creatures, smooth-skinned and red-eyed, rise to the surface and call to her. She understands their cries as they mate, give birth and die. Stars burst above her like celestial fireworks, and her skin crackles with electricity. She leaps into the waves. But just as her toes touch the water, the ocean dries up before her eyes, and the desert explodes in fire around her. The sparks clear and for a moment, there is nothing but an electric, cosmic pause, like the moment before a lightning strike. Then her earthly body floats away like ashes carried on the wind. She merges with the light, her ego dropping away. She is still coming, waves of orgasm wracking her body. She writhes and bucks on the table, as if she were trying to break free of shackles.

As quickly as it happens, it's over.

She sobs in Michael's arms, her tears mixing with his. He strokes her hair. Finally, she opens her eyes. They hold each other in silence. Thoughts come to mind, and she discards them. They seem coy, trivial, as unneeded as shoes on a warm beach. They are remnants of the part of her that would make jokes about what has just happened. But now, she has no need.

"I saw things," she says finally. "Everything was light. I was the light. I saw how it was all connected, and how I was connected to it. I can't explain."

"I know."

When she is ready, he helps her from the table, and wraps her in her robe. They walk hand in hand to their room and she crawls into bed, slipping beneath the white, cool sheets. Later, she will be hungry, but now, she needs to rest.

Michael goes to close the curtains.

"Don't," she says. "I want to see the mountains."

They both know that she can't see the mountains in the darkness, except as indistinct shapes that begin where the stars end. But she knows that they're there, beyond the desert, and for now, that is enough. Their indigo presence burns in her heart.

TANTRIC EXPERIENCE

Orgasmic Third Eye Opening

THE THIRD EYE ORGASM TECHNIQUE IS NOT ABOUT MAKING up fantasies or watching mental movies. This is a meditation; a tantric meditation on the light within.

Though this light may be difficult to see during conventional meditation, the tantric advantage is that the supercharged energy of your sexual climax can burst right through the gates of heaven—the pleasure centers in your brain—and illuminate them. The worst that can happen to you is that you will have a fabulous orgasm!

You are surrendering to your inner light. This light is already there. You don't create it. You discover it. It is the clear light in your mind that illuminates your fantasies. It is the background light source to the movies in your mind's eye.

It may help to think back to any past experience involving light. Perhaps it was a sunrise or sunset at the beach. What about drug experiences? Meditation moments? Vivid dreams?

The classic yoga meditation approach is to gaze at a candle flame, then close your eyes and see that flame in your forehead at the third eye. This ancient strategy is called *tratak*. Most yoga books with a section on meditation teach it.

When you roll your eyes back into your head, this is not just a physical act. It is an inner gesture, a caress upon your brain, and with it you encourage an emotional yielding to subtle, inner ecstatic feeling.

I call this letting-go "swooning." The physical eye movements begin the gesture. They are the trigger, like flicking the switch on your wall that turns on the light. You pick up the flow from there emotionally, intuitively, kinesthetically, and fall backwards deep within.

The key always to red hot tantra is relax, easy does it, be comfortable. It is a mistake to push and push. Instead, relax into your natural ground of being. Explore it and enjoy it more and more. It is already there. It is waiting for you.

Once in place, your eyes stay rolled back. They stay put. Not rigidly or painfully so, but firmly right there. They are locked in place. The light is more easily seen, it is stimulated and provoked in this way.

With the eyes rolled back, it is like the camera has turned back to look at itself. You are going very deep within—you may even feel like you are going, going, gone!

Have you ever pushed on your eyeballs with your fingers? These glowing phosphemes are something like what you may see with this Tibetan Eye Roll technique when you climax. Perhaps you want to start with the clove oil. Dab it on your forehead using the tip of the little finger. Not much is needed. The essential oil is strong.

Roll the eyes up and back. Drink in the delicious burning sensations from the clove oil. The advantage of clove oil is that these sensations last a long time.

You've watched fireworks on the Fourth of July. It is the same with the third eye. When the orgasmic kundalini energy goes up, you will see flashes of light. Do not be concerned with how that will happen. Just be in place. To see the fireworks, you need a good spot. The third eye is that spot. Station your attention there and wait.

To fulfill your third eye love tryst together, you need to let your partner serve you as you do this meditation. Third Eye Orgasm is totally centered on self. To go deep within, you must center on yourself. You must go deep within to see, feel, know who you are—your deep, true self. At first, this may seem selfish, but it evolves into total self-fulfillment. By resting in pure being the innate wholeness is found.

This experience of combining the Tibetan Eye Roll with the sexual climax is very powerful, very pure, very spiritual. It expands on the momentum from your sensual energies. The only sacrifice you make is one of attention—to lift your eyes to your vast mental skies and keep them on the shining prize!

During a private interview, Jeannine of Portland, Oregon, told me "I saw a white light. It became brighter and brighter. I went into the center of it and disappeared. Ever since, life has been much easier for me. It was an experience of enlightenment."

After a workshop, Steve from Seattle, Washington, shared that "I saw rainbows. I felt like I was flying over them. It almost seemed like I left my body. But I never felt scared. There was always an ecstatic feeling that filled me up, that kept my mind quiet and serene."

Stephanie of Los Angeles, California, sent this report to me: "I saw a river of liquid fire go up my spine. It felt incredibly blissful. When the sexual climax occurred, it was almost an afterthought. I felt so complete, so filled, it was like I was in a state that was beyond orgasm, or was the deeper source of the orgasm."

You will have the experience that is right for you. There is nothing more personal than the joyful awakening of this mystical healing energy within you.

Red tantra says "Allow your body to awaken like an innocent sensual child in celebration." Let go! Surrender to the wisdom of Mother Nature exploding intimately within your body as the power of life-force kundalini. If you do not force it, but yield in love and joy instead, you will rise effortlessly higher and higher in consciousness, riding waves of love, light, bliss, and peace.

When you do the Third Eye Orgasm, you are in deep meditation. It is most sacred. It is blissfully effective, yet effortless. This is red tantra meditation!

In the story, Carrie and Michael awaken the primal power of inner light. They blend the love gift of a sensual massage with clove oil and the Third Eye Orgasm. Carrie receives Michael's magical touch. Her orgasmic vision is an earthy scene of electrical release that conveys deep tantric knowledge and empowerment. Carrie realizes "I was the light."

You, too, are the light. Do Third Eye Orgasm. Discover this for yourself.

TANTRIC TALE

Fire Woman

IMAGINE MY SURPRISE WHEN THE PHONE RINGS, AND IT'S BRENT. Almost six months have passed without any word from him. No call. No e-mail. And certainly none from me. I hate playing games, but I hate humiliating myself even more. I'm trying to change old habits. I've been trying not to obsess over men and instead, I've been focused on developing my inner self, et cetera. I've been going to yoga every day, and meditating, and taking lots of hot baths and all that crap. I've even started painting again.

All to try to forget him.

To forget his soft lips and how they played with mine before traveling down my body and between my legs. To forget his tongue, which never seemed to tire. To forget his broad shoulders, still muscular from years of rowing, even ten years after he graduated from college. To forget how his firm butt felt under my hands as I pulled him into me. To forget three nights of the best sex I've ever had, of laughing and talking until dawn.

And I've almost succeeded in forgetting when he calls, as though we had spoken only yesterday. "Hey, Michelle. It's Brent."

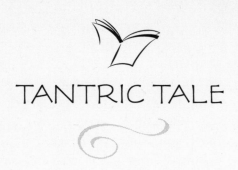

"It's been a long time," is all I can manage. I pull a long lock of hair from behind my ear and twirl it around my finger. It's a bad habit that only gets worse when I'm anxious. And Brent makes me anxious. He doesn't respond. "Are you still there?"

"Of course. I'd like to see you."

I feel my face tingle, and I feel myself grow warm and soft between my legs. I mentally kick myself in the ass. Why is it he produces this reaction in me?

"Oh? What did you have in mind?"

"I can't tell you on the phone."

"Then I'm hanging up."

"If I did tell you what I have in mind, you might be offended. Or scared. So could I come over, and tell you in person instead?" His tone suddenly sounds serious. This throws me.

"I guess."

"I've been thinking about you a lot."

I want to pop back with something smart, like *Oh, you could have fooled me.* But I try to remember everything I've learned in meditation class. *That's anger I'm feeling. Interesting.* I let it go and take a deep breath.

"I see," is all I allow myself.

Brent shows up with two bottles of Merlot from my favorite winery and an expression on his handsome, chiseled face that I haven't seen before. He's always been a self-confident guy, which is what attracted me to him, but now that self-confidence has changed. Matured. I almost want to call it. Serene. He's dressing differently, too. Before, he dressed to show his body, with tight-fitting shirts that defined gorgeous pecs and biceps toned by hours in the gym. Tonight, he wears a plain T-shirt and a clean-but-well-worn pair of Levis. He hugs me tightly.

"It's good to see you," he whispers into my ear.

I pull away from him and begin twirling my hair. "You could have seen me a lot sooner."

"Actually, I couldn't have."

I take the bottles to the kitchen. "What, did you have to leave town?"

"In a matter of speaking."

"You're being very mysterious."

"I had to do some work on myself."

"You make it sound like a construction project." I begin, out of habit, to open the first bottle.

"In a way, it was. Say, let's wait to open the wine. Do you have any herbal tea?" I must look alarmed, because he laughs. "I just want to be present. I want us both to be present."

I put my hand on his forehead as if feeling for a temperature. "Who are you? What have you done with Brent?"

He laughs. "He's right here."

"That's what I'm afraid of." I light the kettle. *What is going on?* I think. I don't trust him. As I prepare the tea, I decide to change the subject, asking him about some mutual friends. Finally, though, my curiosity gets the better of me.

"So, to what do I owe this pleasure?" I ask. I set the pot of tea and two cups on the coffee table and sit next to him on the couch, making sure to leave a full cushion of space between us.

He takes my hand and strokes it as if he were trying to calm a nervous racehorse. My heart begins to race. "I really have been thinking a lot about you. And I'm sorry I didn't call before. I was starting to fall for you, and I knew I wasn't ready."

"C'mon, Brent. You can be more original than that."

"This isn't a line, Michelle. I wasn't the person I wanted to be for you. Look, I know you're on a spiritual path as well, so I'm going to jump right in. When I met you, I was just about to take my own practice to another level. My old way of life—the partying, the drinking, the sleeping around—was killing me. I felt like I was living two lives. So I just had to drop out of the scene for a while. And yes, I did leave town. I went on a one-month meditation retreat."

"You could have let me know, instead of just disappearing."

"I know. I was a jerk. Maybe I was afraid you'd try to talk me out of it. But that's no excuse for hurting you."

My God, he's not kidding, I think, and I feel my heart begin to reach out to him again. He begins telling me about his experiences—about feeling that the layers of his ego were being peeled away, about feeling like for a moment, he could see his true being. *Yes, that's what I want, too,* I think. And there have been times, brief flashes, where I've seen glimpses of what he's describing.

"I need some time to digest all this," I say. "It's going to take some time for me to trust you again."

"I understand."

"Can I open the wine now?"

"Let's save it for next time."

Next time. I know what that means with Brent. It means I won't see him for at least three weeks.

But Brent calls me the next day, and asks if we can get together later in the week. I'm astonished, but I agree. Again, he glides into my apartment on a pillow of serenity. And again he asks only for herbal tea. I pummel him with questions about his little "retreat." If there's a hole in this story, I'm going to find it.

And then he mentions tantra. I can't help it. I burst out laughing.

"I knew this was just a new technique for seduction."

"Tantra is not seduction, Michelle, any more than yoga is just a way to get a better body." He seems almost angry, which surprises me. "It's about spirituality. I know you're skeptical. But hear me out."

He begins describing the difference between white tantra, the masculine form of tantra, and red tantra, the feminine, female-oriented form, based on ancient goddess traditions. And something in me wakes up. Something tells me, *It's okay. Just go for it.*

"But why are you telling me all this? Why did you call me after all these months?"

"There's something about you, Michelle. I felt a strong connection with you. So strong it frightened me. And it wasn't just sexual. I've done a lot of tantric work on my own, but it's something that one has to experience with a partner. And I realized that I wanted that partner to be you."

I make a sudden decision. If this is just a line, I don't care: It's working. I haven't been with another man in six months. *Hell,* I think, *maybe this time I can dump him,* even though I know I'll do nothing of the sort. I lean forward and kiss him. He kisses me back, his tongue playing with mine. I imagine that tongue between my legs, and I moan softly.

"Why me?" I say finally. "I don't know anything about tantra."

"Don't worry. Shiva said that 'your body will understand it long before your mind can put words to it.'"

"I think my body is ready to understand." I pull him down onto me.

We kiss and he begins to grind his pelvis into mine. I wrap my legs around him. I feel his erection and know that I'm already wet. I don't know how he does it, but in one move, he slides off the couch and lifts me up, my legs still wrapped around him. He carries me to the bedroom, and we fall onto the bed. He undresses me slowly, as if he were unwrapping a present. When I'm naked, he runs his hands over my skin, looking at every inch of my body.

"You look like you've never seen a woman before."

"I feel like I haven't. I haven't slept with anyone since the last time we were together."

I stare at him. The old Brent would never have been able to go three days without sex, much less six months. And if he had, he would have already pulled on a condom and slapped on some lube, and we'd be going at it without any foreplay. I reach for him and slip his T-shirt over his head. I unbutton his jeans and slide them over his hips. Then his underwear. His erection is huge, but as I lean in to take it in my mouth, he stops me.

"You first."

He begins kissing my skin, starting with my neck and then working his way over my collarbone, then my breasts. He sucks on my nipples until I'm ready to scream, because by then, his hand is already playing with the hard button between my soft folds. He kisses my stomach, my thighs, and then his tongue is between my legs, replacing his fingers. I can't help it. I begin moaning. He lifts his head.

"Don't stop."

"I just wanted to tell you to breathe."

I obey. As his tongue begins again, I try to steady my breathing and feel the sensations he's producing in my body. He slips one finger into me and begins to vibrate it. I feel my muscles stiffen. I'm speeding to an orgasm—faster than I ever have before—when he stops. I look at him in surprise.

"Keep breathing," he tells me, as he pulls a condom out of his jeans.

It's the same old Brent, but with a little more foreplay than usual, I think, and then I push the thought out of my head and keep breathing. He pulls me on top of him into a sitting position, his legs crossed under him. I gasp as he enters me. It feels unbelievably good. He begins to rock his pelvis gently, so that his pubic bone rubs against my sex. He grabs my butt and holds me against him.

"Keep breathing," he whispers in my ear. "Imagine a blazing light, burning away your fears."

He's starting some sort of rhythm, and I join him. Somewhere in my mind, I realize that I'm entering a place I've only been during meditation. I close my eyes; the light becomes a flame, the flame a conflagration. It illuminates the darkness in my heart, the dark, dank places where my fear, my anxiousness, and my sadness live. I imagine every hurt and every resentment like deadly mushrooms poisoning the well of my soul. The fire burns them all away.

An image comes to me. A woman is dancing around a fire, then through it, in it. She is covered in blood. As she turns toward me, I see insanity in her laughing eyes. *She has killed and eaten my craziness,* I think. *She has eaten both of us.* I shudder, but I also begin moving faster and faster, as if I'm dancing with her. Brett takes one hand that is cupping my butt and with his middle finger, touches the secret rosebud there. I'm so wet and slippery that he easily slides the tip of his finger in. It sends me over the edge.

I realize that I am coming. The orgasm begins in my clitoris and lights me up, traveling up into my womb, then my heart. I feel it exploding out the top of my head. One part of me realizes that I am screaming, and that he is coming, too. But neither of us stops our rhythm. Our orgasms seem to go on and on. Finally, we collapse into each other and tumble onto the bed. He is still inside me, still hard.

Finally, I can breathe. "Brent, I saw something."

"I know. I saw her too. It was Kali, the goddess of fire. The Queen of Kundalini. I knew I'd see her with you." He laughs as if he knows how ridiculous it sounds.

A final shudder, a remnant of the orgasm, courses through me like an aftershock. I don't doubt him.

"You have an old soul, Michelle. Don't be so afraid of it."

Usually, I would be frightened by how well he knows me. Now, I simply listen to him. And then I say exactly what I think. "That's why I joke so much. I've been afraid that I would be too intense for people. And you know, I'm tired of people saying I'm too sensitive. That's who I am."

"That's why I love you."

"Excuse me?" Every nerve ending in my body begins to tingle.

"I love you. I always have. Don't think. Just answer."

It's so ridiculous. This man I've slept with three—now four times. I'm breaking my own rules about keeping men at arm's length before I get too involved. But my rules, the scripts that I've written for my life, burned in the fire.

"I love you, too."

"Good. Let's open the wine now."

We pull apart almost reluctantly. But it's only then that I realize that I'm starving. We fix a plate of fruit and cheese, open the wine, and crawl back into bed. As we sip the Merlot, I feel the joy well up in me. Tomorrow morning, will I regret this? Perhaps. But in the moment when I told Brent I loved him, I was myself, and it felt wonderful.

"What are you laughing about?" Brent asks me.

"You must think I'm easy."

"I think you love sex. Because you love connection."

"Connecting with you."

We eat and drink in comfortable silence, put the plates aside, and fall asleep, spooned into each other as though we were born to sleep that way. In the morning, as the sun is rising, I wake up and I turn to Brent. He's already awake, watching me with a smile.

"It's so easy for me to fall asleep with you," he says. "I feel like I've come home. And yes, I meant what I said last night. I love you."

As I kiss him, morning breath and all, I realize that I have literally burnt a bridge, a bridge to my past life. My past life of fear, fear that there would never be enough—enough money, enough nourishment, enough love. The fire burnt it all away. I'm embarking on a new adventure. I am full of abundance, and full of joy that I never thought possible. I fall asleep again, peaceful at last. I, too, have come home.

TANTRIC EXPERIENCE

Kali Fire Ritual

THE VISUALIZATION OF THE ALL-CONSUMING FIRE OF erotic love is ancient. In sacred tantric worship in India today, the guru sits with his or her consort in the center of a circle of student couples. I believe that fire may have been the first tantric guru.

I may have seen, in a vision I had in 1996, the first tantric circles. Ten thousand years ago, couples sat scattered around a huge bonfire. The fire, a source of wonder to them, was guiding them with its heat, light, sound, and movements.

As they stared into the dancing blaze, listened to the crackling, and felt the seductive warmth, they entered a relaxed, sensuous dreamlike trance. Imagination was set free. The inner flame was ignited. They reached for each other to expand and share the glow of already flowing pleasure.

Images of the flames danced in their minds. They made love with the heat and abandon of the orange-red flames raging and roaring a few feet away.

In tantra, fire is a symbol for sacrifice, for going all the way, for living in the heat that is felt when the ego, which always seeks control, is burned up and surrendered. It is a symbol for the teacher, who brings light and dispels darkness.

Fire also represents kundalini, the mystical heat in the body. When aroused, it rises up the spine. It is said to move in the sinuous style of a snake or the wavelike dance of flames. Kundalini is the source of orgasm's pleasure and of its power to elevate and illuminate. For more on kundalini, see Red Hot Resources, at the back of the book.

You and I were cautioned against playing with fire as children. The same advice applies to the sexual fire for adults. Lovers want to be hot. They want to be on fire for each other. They want to sizzle with lust and light up with electricity.

Yet so many end up getting burned by this mysterious fire. Sexual fire, like physical fire, needs a container. Find a discipline that you enjoy—fire sacrifice, mantra, visualization, ritual, breath meditation, mindful focus on body sensations—and make that your container. Keep it simple. Be consistent. Once you have found it, stay with that one thing.

The visualization of the all-consuming fire is simple and powerful. This fire meditation is associated with Kali, the Dark Goddess of India. She is the Queen of Kundalini, the inner spiritual fire energy behind the blaze of pleasure at orgasm, as well as the lasting brightness of enlightenment.

Kali is universally agreed to be the tantric goddess par excellence. She is the dark, inscrutable patron queen of the red tantra mysteries and has been its guiding light for many thousands of years. She represents female sexuality in its wildest and most liberated state, claiming its birthright of unbounded pleasure without respect for male laws or limitations.

Kali is also renowned for her ability to eat up bad karma. It is said that she is always hungry for your negative energy. Remember anger that smoldered inside of you? What about fear that froze you? Or confusion that overwhelmed you? To her, those energies were bonbons. She *loves* your shit!

The fire meditation is done late at night, at the zenith of the "midnight sun." There are three parts: purification, action, and contemplation.

If you want to just do the sacrificial purification step, you can. If you want to just do the orgasmic action step, you can. If you want to just do the contemplative afterglow step, you can. If you want to do them together, great!

Kali's worship is not rigidly formulated. Spontaneity and authenticity are prized most of all. The process begins with the purification of the tantrika. This first step is quite simple. Just throw whatever is bothering you into the fire, to be burned up and released forever from you.

You can make a real fire, but you don't have to do so. The light of a small red candle will do fine. Or it can all be done with visualization.

The ritual becomes a little more dramatic, which may make it more effective for you, if the problem you wish to be released from is first written down on a piece of paper and then burned. If you want to do this, write boldly with black ink on bright red paper. Black and red are her colors. A small piece of paper will do.

Write your request on one side, such as "Mother Kali, please release (your name here) from (the problem in a few words) with the fire of your grace." Then fold it over and write "KALI, HELP ME" in big letters on the top of it.

Repeating Kali Ma's name, seed sound or mantra sentence (see below), place the paper in the candle flame until it starts to burn. Then put it on a plate or in a bowl that you have set aside for this purpose. Watch it burn to ashes as you continue to repeat her sacred sound.

If it does not burn completely, expose it to the flame again. Repeat, if necessary, until the red paper is burned to black or gray residue and ash.

For her sacred sound, many tantrikas like to repeat the seed mantra "Krim" (pronounced "kring" or "cream"). A seed mantra is a single syllable of condensed power said to contain the essence of the deity's energy. Feel the sound with your body. The "kring" sound strikes your root power center. You may feel its energy resonating at the tailbone or anus, or possibly in the cervix or prostate.

The sound "cream" is felt more in the chest, perhaps as a growing yearning for a blissful expansion of the heart. In English, this sound has attractive meanings that connote sensual richness, smoothness, and luxury.

Another traditional seed mantra used to connect with Kali in meditation is "Kong" (as in King Kong). If you wish, you can repeat her complete mantra "Om Kang Kalika Namahah." Sounded out, this is "Om Kong Kah-lee-ka Nah-ma-ha!" Ideally, this mantra is spoken out loud with passionate enthusiasm.

Or just repeat "Kali Ma, Kali Ma, Kali Ma" softly with sincerity and humility, perhaps as a prayer. She will hear you. She is always listening.

Finally, her name is itself a mantra. Say "Ka-Li" loudly. Pronounce it as two separate syllables: "Kah! Lee!"

Say "Ka" with a low, almost guttural voice. Render the "Li" as a high-pitched sound.

You may sense that the "Ka" awakens your solar plexus center. You may notice how the "Li" sound opens the top of your head, activating your crown center.

If you are not feeling these impacts, perhaps you need to punctuate the sounds more. Focus on the solar plexus and growl the "Ka." Feel the top of your head and sing the "Li."

In essence, this way of pronouncing her name activates the kundalini energy and starts it moving up to the highest center. At the very least, you are likely to feel physically energized and mentally clear after just a few vigorous repetitions.

The action portion is sexual climax. The intensity of the orgasm is experienced as a cleansing fire, burning away ignorance, selfishness, and fear. In the climax, the sacrificial "mahamudra" (great gesture) of no-mind is attained. This kiss of grace from Kali is enhanced by your sincere efforts to surrender to it and remain awake within it. In her role as the wisdom goddess of sex, kundalini, and orgasmic release, Kali has asked me many times to remind tantrikas that a sublime transmission of the Most High takes place at that primal moment.

A male tantrika may visualize his lover as Kali Ma. A female tantrika may visualize herself as Kali or another form of the Goddess. Or she can simply surrender to her senses and feelings. Either way, she will bring the blessings of the Goddess to the embrace.

In solo practice, the visualization is the same. You either are the Goddess or you are united with the Goddess. Since the sensations from sexual and sensual interaction must be created via vivid fantasy, feel free to exaggerate the images, to move your body and breathe as if aroused.

If you are the Goddess, you can choose a partner or not. One female tantrika told me a male angel visited her while doing this ritual meditation. "I shall never forget his great white wings," she said, "as he made love to me."

As arousal builds, see everything—your bed, your bedroom, your home, your city, the earth and, finally, the universe—going up in flames and burning to nothingness. At the moment of climax, see the heat and flames and light reach their ecstatic peak in a cosmic explosion that consumes the universe in one great flash. All of the stars, all at once, go supernova together. In *The Bhagavad Gita,* Krishna, the Hindu Christ, describes the universal self that lives in every heart as looking like "the light of a thousand suns."

Success brings a vision of the universe as a luminous, transparent ocean of blissful light. The cosmic fire boils everything down to the bright, pure, clear essence, where all is one exactly as it is. The great Hindu sage Sri Ramakrishna, the famous Kali devotee who rekindled the worship of Kali in modern times, describes a similar vision as the turning point in his own spiritual life.

Now close with the contemplation stage. Linger in the afterglow. Keep your eyes closed and your body still. Allow your mind to be silent. You may see colors or visions, spontaneously enter higher states of consciousness, receive messages, or otherwise be guided at this time.

In meditation, the tantric queen Kali once said to me: "No-thought is the best sacrifice, not words. The silence of the motionless mind is my ultimate mantra." If you wish, hold each other. Turn your cuddling into an asana, a yoga posture. Once you have entered into it, remain still. Melt into the subtle energetic resonances created by the pulsating, musical interplay of your mutual passions. Allow the peace of the afterglow to pervade your oneness.

After intense practice such as this, enter the world slowly. Take a long hot shower. Give each other massages. Leisurely share an earthy, substantial meal. Specifically, do *not* drive a car immediately after this kind of experience.

These fruits may extend into your daily life, giving you the healing release that you requested of the tantric goddess of change and death. Remember, the death or end of something you *don't* want, such as illness, addiction or poverty, is the birth or new beginning of something you *do* want in your life.

Of course, it may not appear in the exact form that you were picturing!

You are dealing with a great goddess. She reserves the right to have the last word. I know from my own experience that, even when the changes make no sense, she knows what she is doing. It always turns out for the best.

Expect nothing. Receive everything with a smile. You have a new friend. Kali. Think about it. You don't want something? Give it to her. She wants your junk. She is a spiritual recycling center. She processes your personal garbage and converts it to the pure gold of consciousness.

At the very least, your load will be a little lighter now.

In the story, enthusiastic red tantrikas Brent and Michelle identify with the natural spontaneity of the flames. So total is their identification, their meditation, they become that spontaneity–and nothing else is needed. Surrendering to the sweet wonder of sexual ecstasy, they are swept away into a realization of the basis of life, love, sex and soul as bliss, as the raw sweet rush of aliveness.

Erotic spiritual fire burns away their fears and attachments. A flash of illumination follows, revealing the courage to embrace freedom. They trade their boring, predictable future with its dry, cardboard certainties for a more joyful life of living in love together.

As Brent and Michelle discover, spontaneity is the highest yoga.

In the words of the great modern sage Nisargadatta Maharaj, the source for the contemporary spiritual classic *I Am That,* "What is spontaneous, is true. What is true, is spontaneous."

You may not end up a millionaire following this supreme tantric wisdom, but wherever you walk, you will be showered by flowers.

TANTRIC TALE

Unguarded Moment

We are lying in bed. The dishes are put away, the bills paid, the computers turned off. This is my favorite time of day, when you and I lie face to face, and kiss, and talk. Tonight we talk about sex, mostly because we are too tired to have it. You say you want to hear my darkest fantasies, and I pause. I have only one. I hate it, but it is as reliable as my mother's old Ford station wagon for getting me where I want to go. Maybe if I tell it to you, it will disappear.

Here it is.

You have invited several of your friends, all men, to our home. Several hours before they arrive, you prepare me.

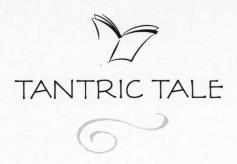

You bring me into the bathroom, which is illuminated by the glow of twenty—exactly twenty—fragrant candles. In my fantasy, our bathroom is expansive and white and marbled, not tiny and cramped as it is in real life. I sit on a saffron-colored cushion on a golden bench and watch as you pour lavender salts under the tap. Then you help me into warm, scented water. With a loofah you smear a fragrant scrub, redolent of apricot and coconut, onto my skin, buffing it until it reddens and glows. You cup your hands into the water and rinse me off, then lather a washcloth with a bar of honey soap and scrub every inch of my body, first massaging my neck and shoulders, then working the lather over my breasts and stomach and even between my legs. Especially between my legs. You spread my knees apart slightly so you can reach my lower lips. You clean me completely. I am as soft and bare as a young girl, because you required, earlier in the day, that I wax completely. You wrap the washcloth around your finger and press it inside me. Leaning me back, you slide your hand under me and wash between my butt cheeks.

Rinsing me again, you help me from the tub, engulfing me in a large snowy bath sheet. You blot the moisture from my skin, not missing a single spot, and anoint me with perfumed oil. I glow. You dry my hair, brushing it to a golden sheen. You blacken my lids with smoky eyeshadow and line my eyes with a black kohl pencil. You rouge my cheeks, dab on bright scarlet lipstick. Finally, you draw a transparent black gown over my head. I am ready. You lead me into our living room and help me into a reclining position on a blood-velvet chaise lounge. In my fantasy, our living room is delivered of its mish-mash of furniture, books, and CDs. Instead, it resembles nothing so much as the salon of a decadent French lord in a secret chateaux, the walls the color of burgundy, heavy curtains blocking the light of a full moon.

The men begin to arrive. There are about ten of them. Some are dark-haired, some are blonde, but they are, to a man, as perfect as ancient Greek statues. My only job, now, is to offer myself up as an object for their gaze while they drink and play cards.

They do not look at me. I know they notice me, appreciate me, but I might as well be a statue. Only you see me, and every so often, as you move among them, you smile at me. I can't tear my eyes from your gaze. The truth is, I am afraid to look at the men. I sense the energy growing in the room.

Finally, it is time. You kneel between my legs and bestow a kiss on my lips, your tongue soft and insistent. But when I reach up to touch you, you roughly move my hands back to the arms of the chair. You move your mouth down my body and push up the hem of the gown to display my sex. You move your mouth onto my clitoris, spiraling your tongue round and round. The men stare. Shame flows through me, but I can't help but respond to your tongue. My hips begin to rock against your mouth. You reach up and begin to play with my nipples until they protrude.

I am wet, so wet that when you take your hand from my nipple, you can easily slide two fingers deep inside me, thrusting them in and out. They hint at what you'd like to do to me with your hardness. Soon, you sense that I am approaching orgasm. You pull your fingers out, and touch the entrance to my anus. Your fingers are so slick that they slide in to the first knuckle. My legs stiffen, my toes pointing straight out. My stomach tightens. You move your tongue faster and faster until I come. In the fantasy, that is. In real life, as I'm having this fantasy, I've only just begun to get aroused.

"Only sluts get so aroused in front of strange men," you whisper. "Only sluts come in front of strangers." You tear the nightgown in half as though it were gossamer.

This is the sign. The men disrobe, revealing smooth, muscular torsos and defined abs. They are already hard.

I try to get up, but some of the men have already moved around me. The fantasy varies depending on how I'm feeling: Sometimes they fasten my arms to the chair with handcuffs, and the metal digs into my flesh; in other versions of the fantasy, they use bondage tape or scarves. Sometimes four men surround me, two men holding my wrists while the other two hold my legs apart. They laugh at my fear. They grab my hair and paw at my breasts.

I realize that one of the men has won the opportunity to be the first to initiate me. His manhood is the biggest, and I struggle as he approaches the chair, but to no avail. He enters me without preamble. Even though I'm slick from coming, I feel as though I've been cloven in two. You stand behind me, holding my hair, as he pounds against me without mercy.

"Go ahead," you say. "Take all of it." Sometimes you turn my head and let me suck you as the stranger has his way with me. But sometimes, you beckon over another man, and force me to suck him.

After the first man finishes, the others take turns. Two of them ask you if they can take me together, and you agree. They release me from my restraints and turn me onto my hands and knees. One lies back on the couch and forces me to suck him as the other enters me from behind after giving my butt a few rough slaps. After a while, the two men switch positions. Every man there gets a shot at me. If I try to struggle, they laugh.

At this point, I barely need the fantasy anymore. I only need one more image to make myself come.

When each of the men except you has had me, it is time for the second part of the initiation. You lie me on my stomach and put a large pillow under my hips. You spread lube between my butt cheeks. I realize what's coming: You are going to let these men have my other, more secret entrance, one by one. And this is enough to make me come, hard, bucking against my own hand as I stroke myself madly.

I am no longer facing you. I lie on my back, staring at the ceiling. But I'm aroused. I can't help touching myself. Even in telling you, I've become wet.

"I hate this fantasy," I tell you. "I can't believe I let my guard down and told you."

"Why?"

"Even when I'm with you, I have to use it." What I don't say is that I know you like to watch me come, and I'm afraid that this is the only way I can do it. But the fantasy separates me from you. It separates me from my body. It separates me from myself.

You listen. To my surprise, you don't seem shocked. In fact, when I look over at you, I can see that you are as aroused as I have been in the telling. You slide your fingers between my legs and dip them into my wetness. You lick my wetness from your fingers.

"What are you thinking?" I ask. I want you so badly.

"Something Jung said. 'Everyone carries a shadow.'"

"What does that mean?"

"If you don't bring it to light, it'll keep tripping you up. Like a log at the bottom of a river that you keep snagging your boat on."

I laugh. "The problem with fantasies is that if you actually do them, they lose their power. So I'm not letting you offer me up to ten of your friends."

"That's not what I'm saying." You get up from the bed and begin to light the candles on our bedside table, then a jasmine-scented candle on our dresser. Flickering light fills the room, and I feel as though I'm floating. You light the candles in the wall sconces opposite our bed. I admire your long torso, your powerful butt and legs. Your olive skin appears golden in the flickering candlelight. "How do you feel, now that you've told me the fantasy?"

"I don't know. Better, in a way."

You take something out of the dresser and come back to the bed. I see that you're holding several of my silk scarves, one of them wrapped around something. I know that it is one of my vibrators.

You kiss me. "Tonight is going to be all about you."

You lean me back on the sheets and move my hands above my head. You tie them to each other, and then tie one end of the scarf to the bed frame, but the scarf is tied so loosely that I know I could slip my hands out if I wanted. Then you blindfold me with another scarf.

I am excited, but frightened. "What if I can't come?"

"If you can't, you can't. This isn't a performance. Your only job is to feel sensations. Don't think, don't fantasize. Just feel."

I am absolved. You stroke my skin with sandalwood-scented massage oil. You kiss and suck my nipples. You kiss my chest, my stomach, my belly button. You gently spread my legs and kiss the soft skin of my inner thighs. You move up, and soon your tongue works its way between my soft folds.

The blood-velvet chaise comes back for a moment, but I push it away. I breathe and focus on the feel of the sheets against my skin and your tongue against me. *If I can't come, I can't come.* But my breath quickens.

You turn me over so that I'm on my forearms, my butt in the air. You put a pillow under my hips and push me down against it. You turn the vibrator to a low hum and slide it under me, where it thrums against me. I hear you take something from the nightstand and open the bottle of lube. I feel a slight pressure against my anus and realize that I'm feeling the plug that has gone unused until tonight. Gently, you slide it into me, bit by bit, until its flared body fills me.

The blood-velvet chaise lounge reappears, but I don't push it away. I imagine myself on it, with one of the men behind me, filling me, but this time, I break free of my bonds. The scarves tying me to the chair snap like weak threads, and the man pulls out of me. The men try to hold me down, but I flick their hands away as though they were flies. They are surprised by my strength, aroused by it. The stronger I become, the hotter I am. They jostle each other to get to me, but I shove them away, punch them, kick them, sending them flying to the corners of the room. In my imagination, you watch me, impressed. I jump onto the chair and tower above their bruised, cowering figures. I am an avenging goddess.

"I don't need you," I yell. "We don't need you."

I wave my arms as if to erase them. Leeched of their power, the men dissolve like mist on a warm day. I don't need them, with you here, and us both in control. *If I can't come, I can't come.* But it's okay if I do. It's okay.

As I accustom myself to the plug, you move the vibrator against me. I let myself moan. Then I feel the tip of your penis against my wetness. Waves of pleasure radiate up from my sex. The thought *I can't come unless I'm on my back* pops into my head. *Why not?* I answer myself. I give myself permission to let go.

You pull me up onto my knees, and I slide onto you. I barely notice when my hands come loose from the scarves. I just know that now, I can push against you. With one hand, you hold my hip against yours, while with your other hand, you rub the vibrator against me. I feel like the plug, your hardness, and my clitoris are touching.

Suddenly, I realize that I am on the path to orgasm. Sometimes, just this thought would be enough to drain the pleasure out of me. But I let go. I can't stop the sensations. I brace myself against the bed to push against you harder. It's enough.

"Do it," you say.

And I come and come against you, crying out. We collapse onto the bed. You put the vibrator and plug aside. I don't even know whether you've come. You wrap your arms around me as my breathing returns slowly to normal. The men have long since disappeared into the shadows. I no longer need them, because for now, tonight, you and I are more than enough.

TANTRIC EXPERIENCE

Truth Through Fantasy

FANTASY, EVEN VIOLENT FANTASY, IS HEALTHY! TRUST IS needed. Trust in your erotic dreams and fantasies. Trust in your innate goodness and wholeness. Intense fantasy with sexual release enables you to safely get in touch with your dark, inner forces.

Tantra says: Stop pretending.

These forces are alive inside you right now. Don't judge them. Don't deny them. These primitive energies are buzzing with power that you need. Embrace them and be their loving master. Scientific studies have established that violent sexual fantasies, even if repeated on a regular, long-term basis, do not lead to harm.

Tantra explains it this way: The opposite is the real.

What a person fantasizes about on the outside is what they miss on the inside. A person does not fantasize about what they have. They fantasize about what they don't have, about what they want to have, about the kind of energy that will balance them.

In the dialogue between the surface and the depths, the imagination is the translator, the gatekeeper, the escort. Waking erotic fantasies, like erotic dreams, reveal what is true about us with symbolic pictures, phrases, and story lines.

The tantrika in this story is fantasizing about aggression, about force. It is crude in the story because it is unconscious in her. This is on the surface. Tantra reveals the secret in her depths: She is too passive.

The dream of her soul is to claim her power and be assertive in her daily life. She made love in her erotic fantasies to her inner darkness. She assertively embraced the hidden power of her renegade parts.

A healing, a tantric healing, occurred.

Tantra says the energies have been released, the problem solved, the conflict resolved, all through pleasure, without harming anyone. These coarse, subconscious energies no longer need to be compulsively expressed or repressed.

Nor will she feel depressed. Her dark, dense energies have been lived through, exhausted, burned up, transformed in the safe crucible of her imagination, as if in a dream, as if their sentence was death by delicious orgasm.

The essence of tantra is to trust and embrace the whole self, all of its parts, including that which is ugly to you, that which you don't like, that which frightens you. The freedom of enlightenment is the freedom to be your whole self, unconditionally, spontaneously, all of the time.

The impulsive joys of erotic play and sexual orgasm echo this freedom. They celebrate it with liberating tastes. Tantric sex is the hors d'oeuvre of enlightenment. To enter the mystery of how to live in that freedom, relax. Absorb the wild intuitive wisdom just revealed by the unblocked pleasure flow of your climax.

Float in this living glow as if on a flowing river. Allow thoughts, images, insights to play in your mind. Kiss the sky. Melt into space. Enter the dreamtime.

Take your time. Return slowly, quietly, gently to your body. The afterglow is a form of rebirth. A living intelligence, a kind of magic genie (or genius), permeates all erotic pleasure like a perfume. Ask this consciousness a direct question.

You might as well. You have already rubbed the magic lamp.

"What can you teach me about the art of living? About letting go?"

Let tantra's gift of chaotic symmetry illuminate your being. Let the creative wave force of sexual abandon saturate your body, your mind, your relationships, your work, your heart, your life.

I promise you this: You will never be bored.

TANTRIC TALE

Dream Lover

AT A GOING-AWAY PARTY FOR ONE OF MY HUSBAND'S school chums, we find ourselves trapped in the kitchen by a loud debate about the war. I'm following the progress of a trail of ants across Josie's kitchen counter and daydreaming about the sex that Frank and I had that afternoon when I catch sight of a handsome, light-haired man in glasses waving to me from the ratty couch in the living room. When I realize that he's pointing to a free armchair, I grab Frank's hand and drag him out of the kitchen.

"You guys were in so much pain we had to save you," says our rescuer as we perch on the edge of the armchair. He has bright, blue eyes and blonde hair that sticks up in gelled spikes, and has his arm around a pretty woman with a heart-shaped face and hair that almost matches his. They introduce themselves as Corinne and Sam, and Corinne promptly puts her head on Sam's shoulder. *He's mine*, she seems to be reminding me, though she really doesn't need to. I'm perfectly happy with Frank, my quiet, funny, photographer husband. I reach over and stroke Frank's curly brown hair, just to show Corinne that's I'm not a threat, and she and I exchange smiles.

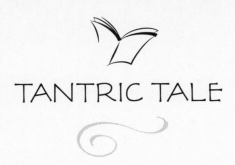

We end up talking to Corinne and Sam until 3 A.M., when a yawning Josie announces she's going to bed. The four of us have discovered that we share identical views on books, politics, and movies. We play off each other perfectly: Sam and I are loud, boisterous, and melodramatic; Corinne and Frank are sly and dry as martinis. No one seems to want us to end the conversation except our hostess.

We whisper our goodbyes in the quiet oak-lined street outside the apartment. The pinkish glow of a streetlamp envelops us. When I give Sam a goodnight hug, I feel like I've met my male twin, the brother I never had. "We'll have to do this again sometime," he says.

And we do. We become inseparable, going to dinner, to movies, on hikes. We are the Four Musketeers. Brothers and sisters. There's no question where the lines are drawn, and no desire to cross them.

Until the night Sam and I go to the movies.

Frank is working late in the darkroom, so Corinne, Sam, and I decide to go see the latest Spike Lee film. Just as I'm about to walk out the door, the phone rings. It's Sam. Corinne has just been struck down by a stomachache; do I still want to go? Sure. Why not.

Halfway through the movie, some guy is about to get beat up. Forgetting that I'm sitting next to Sam and not Frank, I cover my eyes and reach for his hand. As soon as my fingers close around his, I realize my mistake, but it's too late. I have two choices: I can laugh and apologize and snatch my hand away, or I can leave it there. And in that split second of deciding, Sam makes the decision for me, because he closes his fingers around mine and tightens.

I stare at the screen, but I'm no longer able to see what's on it, and my face grows as cold as if I'd just opened a freezer door. Sam slowly caresses my fingers with his thumb. I swell and grow moist in my jeans. If this were a first date, I would guide his hand between my legs so that he could feel the heat.

But I can't. I have to watch the movie, in the dark, our hands intertwined on the red velvet armrest. The more Sam strokes my hand, the wetter I become. When the movie finally ends and the lights in the theater come up, Sam drops my hand and turns to me with a smile.

"That was great," he says. "Do you want to stay for the credits?"

When I get home, I realize that I can't show Frank how wet and aroused I am. So I go into the bathroom, lie on the purple bath rung and masturbate furtively, silently, imagining that it's Sam's penis inside me. I envision that my middle finger is actually Sam's thumb, and when I come, my head snaps back onto the cold tile floor. In the morning, there will be a bump.

That night, I have a dream. I'm in an Italian restaurant in San Francisco, sitting at the bar. The pink marble of the bar feels cold against the bare skin of my forearms; I wish I'd brought a sweater. The pattern of the wallpaper is interlocking pink diamonds, like a harlequin's tunic. The waiters wear black tuxedos. At the end of the bar, an old man in a camelhair jacket talks to a woman with black, pixie-ish hair.

"I never let him answer questions on the stand," the old man says.

Past the old man, I can see out the window to Stockton Street. A sign points the way to Coit Tower. Below it is a stop sign. I realize that Sam is standing outside, looking in at me through the window and smiling. It's then that I realize I'm dreaming.

"Christ, that's so obvious," I say to the bartender. "A stop sign. 'Coit' Tower. Give me a break."

Frank wakes me up. "You were laughing," he tells me.

That weekend, we have dinner at Sam and Corinne's tiny apartment, which looks out over a dry creek bed. When I go outside to light a candle on the patio table, Sam follows me. Our spouses are huddled over the CD rack, picking out background music.

"I had a dream about you the night we went to the movie," Sam says quietly.

I just look at him. I'm afraid to speak.

"I dreamt that I was standing outside a restaurant that I knew was run by assassins," he says. "You were sitting at the bar inside. The door was locked, and I was rapping on the window to get your attention." He starts to laugh. "But you just looked at me and flipped me off!"

My laugh is so loud that Frank and Corinne stop what they're doing.

"What's so funny?" Frank calls.

I dream that night that Sam and I are in a department store buying a birthday present for Corinne. He starts kissing me by the kitchenwares, pressing me up against a display of blenders. I'm afraid that we'll knock the display over, so I drag him over to Linens. He pushes me back onto a bed that's as puffy as a big marshmallow, then pulls off my pants and begins licking me. Curious shoppers crowd around us. Finally, I push him away, pull up my pants, and run to the escalator.

I wake up and look over at Frank, who dozes peacefully on his back. I reach over and stroke him until he's hard and awake. Then I climb on top of him and rock against him until I come.

In the morning he comes up behind me in the kitchen and wraps his arms around my waist.

"I had the best dream last night," he whispers in my ear. "Or maybe, maybe it wasn't a dream after all."

I'm in a booth at Ann's Coffee Shop, taking advantage of the air conditioning and trying to study, when Sam plops down into the seat opposite me.

"I knew you'd be here," he announces.

"I'm always here. I can't get any studying done at home."

"What are you reading?" he says, taking my book from me.

"Women's amatory fiction of the eighteenth century. I have to give a presentation in my seminar next week."

He shudders. "I could never go back to school."

"I sometimes wonder why I am. I must be dreaming if I think I'm going to get a teaching position in this economy."

He studies the cover of the book. "Speaking of dreams, do you want to go with me to buy a birthday present for Corinne? I was thinking of getting her a blender."

I drop my highlighter. He raises his head and looks at me. I notice for the first time that there are circles under his eyes.

"What the hell is going on, Catherine? Should we just go home right now and fuck and get it out of our systems?"

Once again, I become instantly wet. I have an image of our bodies together, naked, and I want to touch myself right there, in the diner, to show him what I look like when I come. "We can't."

"I know. Then stay out of my dreams."

"You stay out of mine!"

"I would if you would just fuck me in the dreams. I'm always following you, and you're always running away. What do you think would happen if I caught you?"

"In the dream?"

"Yes, in the dream."

We stare at each other for what seems like forever. I want to reach for his hand, but I keep it in my lap. Finally, I'm the one to break the silence. "I don't know. But I don't want to ruin what the four of us have."

"Neither do I."

The door to Sam and Corinne's apartment is open when I arrive. Dozens of candles flicker along the windowsill, on the table. No one's in the kitchen of the living room, and I think maybe I've got the wrong night. I walk down the hall to the bedroom. I don't remember the walls being painted this shade of red, or the hall being this long, but I accept it. The walls in the bedroom are bare of any photographs or art. Sam sits at the head of the bed, his knees drawn up to his chest. He wears a T-shirt and a pair of sweatpants, as though he's just come from the gym. I sit next to him.

I turn my head to Sam's, and we begin kissing. His lips are soft, cool; his tongue is just as I imagined it, delicate and insistent.

"I've wanted to do that since the moment I met you." It's a corny thing for him to say, but it's what I want to hear.

We begin to kiss again, and his hands slide under my T-shirt. I wonder to myself why I didn't wear anything sexier. I'm not even wearing a bra. It doesn't matter anyway: Sam pulls my shirt over my head, and I wriggle out of my jeans. Then I undress him. His body is as imperfect and as sexy as I imagined it: I love the paleness of his skin, the love handles at his hips, the slight swell of his stomach.

His penis is long and slender. I take it in my mouth and begin to lick and suck it gently. Soon I feel his mouth on me, his tongue parting my lower lips, nudging my rosebud into hardness. We lay like that, mouth to sex, for what seems like hours. Over and over, he brings me to the edge of orgasm, then lightens the pressure of his tongue.

"I don't want you to come yet," he whispers from between my legs.

Outside, I hear rushing water. Has the creek filled? I think of floods.

"Don't worry," he says. "It's safe."

I pull away from him. "I want you inside me."

I lie so that my head is at the foot of the bed. I spread my legs as far as they will go and brace my hands on the bedposts that have suddenly appeared. Putting his thumb on my clitoris, Sam enters me so slowly that I want to scream. I'm trying hard not to come.

"You're torturing me," I moan.

"I want it to last."

He begins to thrust into me. I raise my knees so that he can enter me more deeply, and I feel him bump against my womb. I begin to see stars. He makes love to me for a while like that, then flips me onto my hands and knees and enters me from behind, pulling my hips against his again and again. Then he slows and puts his fingers back on my swollen button. Waves of pleasure shoot out from my womb.

"I'm getting close," I warn him.

"I want to see your face when you come."

Again, I pull away—it's agony to feel his penis slide out of me—and lie on my back so he can enter me. He licks and sucks my nipples; he slips a hand under the small of my back so that my clitoris grinds against his pubic bone. We thrust against each other faster and faster. The room grows dark around us; Sam's skin seems to glow. *He is literally fucking the living daylights out of me,* I think. His body moves as fast against my hard nub as my own fingers would if I were masturbating.

"Just like that," I whisper. "Just like that."

Suddenly I'm coming, and coming, and I can't stop. The room explodes around me in white light, and the creek becomes a tidal wave that bursts into the room and tumbles us over and over in space. Sam's crying out, too, yelling my name so loudly that I can feel it in my skin.

Frank is shaking me awake. "Catherine!" His eyes, full of worry, search mine. "You're having a nightmare. You're sweating."

"It's okay," I say, pulling him close, wrapping my arms and legs around him. "Everything is okay now."

When I see Sam and Corinne next for Corinne's birthday party, the dreams seem like something that happened a million years before. Corinne, smelling like jasmine, looks beautiful in a low-cut black dress. She giggles like a schoolgirl.

"I've always wanted to come to this restaurant," she gushes, hugging me.

As we follow the hostess to the table where our other friends wait, Sam puts an arm around me and squeezes. "It worked," he says. I nod.

"What?" Frank asks.

"This place. Catherine suggested it. She knew Corinne wanted to come here."

It is the only lie we will have to tell, although in fact, I did pick the restaurant. In this waking life, Sam is once again my friend again, my twin.

TANTRIC EXPERIENCE

Erotic Lucid Dreaming

In concept, dream lucidity is simple. You continue dreaming, yet remain conscious that you are dreaming. In your dreams, you can have fantastic erotic adventures and other ecstatic experiences that are impossible on the physical plane.

You may have more success with lucid dreaming if you set up ideal, peaceful conditions similar to those of a meditation retreat. A dream quest or ritual dream incubation adventure can involve camping out in the wilderness under skies blazing with stars. You can conduct a personal lucid dreaming retreat at home, too. Set aside an evening for dream study, play, and journaling instead of watching television!

Other special, out of the ordinary preparations, such as attending seminars or studying with a lucid dreaming expert or shaman, will probably also help to support greater dream lucidity, clarity, and control. Anything you do that impresses your subconscious mind with the intensity of your commitment to conscious dreaming will help.

Stephen LaBerge's Lucidity Institute offers the NovaDreamer, a proven technology to help you awaken within your dreams and become lucid. If you are serious about lucid dreaming, erotic or otherwise, but aren't having the success you would like, definitely try this device. The Lucidity Institute is the leading dream research center in the world. You will find more information in Red Hot Resources, at the back of the book.

As you explore the erotic possibilities of your dreams, you will discover that your inner dream wisdom forces have much to show you. For example, if you start having recurring dreams about snakes that make you uncomfortable, journal those dreams in detail. These dreams are exposing your sexual inhibitions and telling you how to release them. Weeks, months, even years later, those dreams will continue to divulge valuable insights—another reason to write them down.

Erotic dreams that mix pleasure with pain, and perhaps punishment, may be healing sexual numbness. One woman who was not yet orgasmic had a series of dreams that when her husband approached her to make love, a thick, scratchy fabric covered her pelvic area. She felt a frustrating prickly heat. Embracing the uncomfortable prickly heat sensations in a dream, she realized that childhood conditioning of shame and guilt was literally blanketing her sensations there. Soon after, she was able to achieve orgasms during intercourse with her husband.

Dreams where you are distressed in sexual situations may also point to erotic fantasies or needs that you are reluctant to admit or too shy to request. Again, the message is in the symbols and details. Become a dream detective and decipher your dreams!

Here are some tips for having rewarding, exciting erotic dreams with a tantric, even transcendental flavor. These are the same exact techniques I have used to have fabulous, unforgettable erotic dreams. Working with these techniques sets the stage for lucid erotic dreaming. The more advanced ideas for achieving dream lucidity follow.

- When you wake up, do not move your body. Keep your eyes closed and lie completely still. This will aid your dream recall enormously. Night dreams are like a fragile silken cocoon around the body. If you move suddenly, this filmy substance is broken and quickly dissipates. A dream fully recalled and relived in this motionless "dream afterglow posture" can be as good as a lucid dream.

- Keep a journal close at hand. It can be as simple or fancy as you like. Even writing down bits and pieces of your dream is helpful. Keeping a dream journal is probably the single most useful step you can take to increase your dream power. The better your recall of your dreams, the better your chance of becoming lucid.
- Here is a tantric trick for having sexual dreams. Right before sleep, pleasure yourself very close to orgasm. You can even hump your pillow! Do this for several nights in a row. You will have sizzling erotic dreams!
- Choose the kind of content you would like to have in your dreams that night. Half an hour before going to bed, fill your mind with thoughts and images related to your dream theme. Try watching a movie or documentary about the topic. Films are like prepackaged dreams.
- Dreaming about film, television, and music personalities has its advantages. Since they are already elevated to star status, it is almost as if they already are dream characters in your waking life. An amazing dream encounter with them can be as easy as gazing at their picture during the day and thinking of them as you fall asleep.
- Create an altar or other special spot for your dreamwork journal, pictures, affirmations, books and other tools. It does not have to cover a large area. It can be a corner on your desk at home or work that is completely dedicated to dream theme images, symbols, statues or other dream reminder objects. This impresses upon your subconscious that your dreamwork now has, quite literally, an important *place* in your life.
- Kava kava, melatonin, vitamin C, and Calea zacatechichi (Mexican dream herb) are reported to cause dreams that are vivid and erotic, even lucid, especially when taken about half an hour before bedtime.

- Sleeping pills result in less restful sleep. Alcohol interferes with dream recall. Both tend to prevent lucidity.
- Make a list of erotic experiences you would like to have—or have again! Perhaps you have never made love on a bed strewn with roses. As you fall asleep, imagine a movie in your mind with this scene. Since it is only a dream, you can make it a multimillion dollar production. After all, you deserve to star in a big budget movie with lavish special effects!
- Whether or not you get good at lucid dreaming, you can still have thrilling, amazing sexual dreams that break the rules. Go to orgies, have threesomes, attend masked erotic balls! Make love flying in the air, in rainbow waterfalls, on the planet Venus.
- Try mutual dreaming. One seasoned erotic dreamer tells new female acquaintances "There's a really cool bar on the astral plane. I'll meet you there tonight." His astral trysts are, in his words, "out of this world!"

Here are some ways to encourage dream lucidity. Lucidity is *not* the Holy Grail of dreaming. If lucidity doesn't come easily, don't be concerned. Just like playing piano or doing the mambo, some people have more of a knack for it.

- Look at your hand during the day and ask yourself "Am I dreaming or not?" Do this from five to ten times a day. As this little ritual becomes a habit, it appears in your dreams. When you ask this question while you are dreaming, you may wake up within your dream and become lucid. Try writing the letter "C" (for "consciousness") on your palm. Many people report this little gem is the best lucidity strategy of all.
- As you drift off to sleep, gently repeat to yourself "I will be conscious in my dreams."
- Encourage floating or flying in your dreams. Flying and erotic dream experiences are connected. The feeling of the wind blowing past your face as you do this dream flying is said to trigger blissful erotic dream states.

- Any situation that somehow feels like a dream, moments of intense emotion, instances of déjà vu, strange coincidences or surprising synchronicities can be met with the question "Am I dreaming or not?"
- Encourage the feeling that right now, even in an apparently wide awake state in the so-called real world, you are, in fact, asleep and lost in a dream. Then ask yourself "Am I dreaming or not?"
- Meditate before you go to sleep. The experts agree it aids lucidity.
- If a dream character starts talking to you, give them your full attention and answer them. A dream character engaging you in conversation or offering advice is a reliable sign that you are about to go lucid in your dream.
- Don't avoid frightful objects or entities. Turn around and face them.
- Reread your dreams from your journal. This is especially helpful just before going to sleep.
- Look for repeating themes in your dreams. Dwell on these themes and ask yourself how they are related to your waking life.
- The amazing wealth of dream resources on the Internet includes dynamic dream networks. People are helping each other dream more lucidly and effectively via e-mail communications, forums, and mutual dream projects.

If you are interested in having cosmic orgasm dreams, then run, do not walk, to the nearest bookstore and buy *Pathway to Ecstasy: the Way of the Dream Mandala* by Patricia Garfield, Ph.D. Or order it on the Internet. I don't care. Just get it!

Does it sound like I'm passing the buck here? Maybe I am just a little, but I know what I'm doing. I've been studying dreams for nearly forty years, and Patricia's book is still the one, the only reliable, authentic, truly tantric guide to having orgasmic, mystical dream events.

When her book came out in the 1970s, it was a revelation for me as well as thousands of other readers. She opened an entirely new, unexplored territory for all of us. Up until then, there had been erotic dreams and lucid dreams and message dreams. But there had been no precedent for erotic cosmic mystical enlightenment dreams!

In Red Hot Resources, you will find a link to a revealing interview with Patricia. She talks about her personal approach to erotic lucid dreaming and how she came up with the remarkable spiritual erotic imagery in her book.

When I worked with her book, I began to experience my own version of her cosmic orgasmic dreams. I was a ball of luminous erotic energy that exploded into white orgasmic light. I ecstatically fused with mysterious dream beings. I was a wave in a sparkling ocean of bliss.

Here are a few more suggestions based on my experiences:

- Write in your dream journal a fantasy description of meeting and merging with a beautiful white or gold light that radiates warm, personal, perfect love. This light can be perceived as a ball, pillar or star, as an angel, as a radiant person.
- If you have a dream in which your body is made of light or is a ball of light and you meet another being like yourself, feel free to simply melt with them in an "astral merge" and explode into nameless, faceless bliss. Sex is far more casual on the dream plane. There are no jealous husbands or wives, no diseases, and nobody gets pregnant. In *Journeys Out of the Body,* Robert Monroe describes astral sex sorties where anonymous or group fusions produce more pleasure than physical sex.
- Make up a divine personality that is the unique combination of all the physical, emotional, mental, spiritual, and erotic characteristics you would like in your dream lover—they are gorgeous; they are incredibly loving, generous, and kind; they are a fantastic lover; they are rich, famous and powerful; and they are madly in love with you! Like I said, anything is possible in your dreams!

- When you go to sleep, see your chosen one in your mind's eye. Encourage a yearning in your heart to achieve a perfect, magical meeting with this exciting erotic dream guide. Pray or otherwise talk to them sincerely, asking that they show you the perfect love, light, and bliss that you seek. Ask them to guide you and protect you. Visualize that your dream meeting with them leads to a perfect blending of energies and personalities. This ideal union culminates in a blissful blaze of loving light. You are showered with transcendental gifts.

In Tibetan dream yoga, this benign, divine personality is called a *yidam*. The yidam is visualized as having a glowing white, naked, perfect body. She glows in this way because she is the very essence of the divine light in human form, made personal and available for you.

The dream god/goddess or yidam skillfully combines in an exquisite, compelling living image the magnetic power of sexual attractiveness and the transcendental intimacy of the spiritual light. She is female if you are male, male if you are female. However, same-sex preferences should be honored, as the attractiveness of this figure is key.

Your dream lover, yidam, whether god or goddess, is a teaching figure, a blessed guide, but he or she is not an end in itself. Merging with them in blissful, bright, earthmoving dream orgasms is not the final goal. Beyond images of the human form, even that of ideal, living gods and goddesses, is the perfect, infinite light itself.

Just as pure white light is the source for all the colors of the rainbow, and so for all forms and phenomena, so, ultimately, is this light the source for all dreams, dream events, and dream figures. Only this light can be the final dream destination. Only this light holds the final answers.

In this clear light, paradoxically, is found the end of dreams and the fulfillment of the highest tantric promise—to awaken within this dream called life, and enjoy it as if it is a spontaneous dream. Sex is the beginning of tantra for many, but it need not be the end. In tracing the secret of waking and dream sexual bliss to its central source, the unity within, the answer to everything, and not just sex and dreams, is found.

The pinnacle of lucid dreaming is conscious union with the clear white light of the Source. Separate identity is dissolved in blissful, total fusion with luminous primal reality. The complete melting of the ego feeling into this Light, even in a dream, is an experience of true enlightenment. It is the ultimate spiritual orgasm. You will never forget it. It will change your life. When you return to your waking world, you will know you *are* that wonderful Light.

In the story, Catherine and Sam embark on a series of mutual dream adventures. Spontaneously, they explore the erotic possibilities of their sexual chemistry without violating their committed relationships. Facing each other in waking life, they agree to resolve their ongoing sexual tensions by consummating their desires in a dream. Enriched by the encounter, they successfully eliminate the need for a destructive waking world dramatization. Catherine and Sam show us that there is no limit to the erotic and healing potential of dreams.

CHAPTER SIX

Tantric Hearing

TANTRIC TALE

The Diary of Red Snake Woman

WHEN MY MOTHER FINALLY DECIDED TO SELL HER childhood home in Wyoming and move into a fancy senior citizen's home, the task of going through the attic fell to me. My brothers all had good excuses why they couldn't help, most revolving around work deadlines and childcare. But I knew exactly what was going on. They were afraid of the attic. Over the years, as we'd grown up and moved away, it had become one big storage locker.

That's how I found myself trapped there on a gorgeous May morning, facing the accumulation of fifty years of family life, while my boyfriend Greg wandered the streets of McKinnon in search of a good café. I'd already spent several hours sorting stuff into piles. It was getting close to noon, and I'd totally underestimated the amount of work I had ahead of me. I pulled an old trunk out of one corner to use as a seat while I tried to figure out my next step.

At some point, I looked down at the trunk. I remembered my mom saying that it had belonged to my grandmother, but I had no idea what was inside, so I stood up and lifted the lid. Inside were piles and piles of yellowed papers: letters, tied together with ribbon, old photographs, and documents that looked so brittle I was afraid they'd crumble if I touched them. It would take me hours to sort through everything.

But then something caught my eye: a small book, wrapped in lace. I gingerly lifted it from the faded lining of the trunk and unwrapped it. When I turned to the first page, I realized that it wasn't a book at all: It was a journal. Written on the thin paper in a spidery cursive were the words: *The Diary of Earline Runningwater Stewart.*

I stared at the words in surprise. Earline Stewart, my great-grandmother on my mother's side, had been spoken of only in hushed tones as I was growing up, but I had never been able to get anyone to tell me what was so scandalous about her. And I never knew that her middle name was Runningwater. Could it be that she had Shoshone in her? I turned to the first entry.

> **October 28, 1895.** Today is my eighteenth birthday, and I'm reading the books that Grandpa brought me from back east. I'm going to keep a diary like some of those other ladies. But my diary is going to be different. My diary is going to be real. I'm going to write all those things that no one talks about.
>
> **October 29, 1895.** Papa wants me to find a man and get married. I told him I'm not ready. I don't think he liked that. He asked me which man I liked at my birthday party and I told him I liked them all. I don't think he liked that either.

I smiled. A woman afraid to commit to one man, just like myself. Even after five years, I was still crazy about Greg, but I couldn't explain why I was so reluctant to get married. I turned back to the diary.

> **November 3, 1895.** Guess what, Diary. I'm a woman now. Last night I was layin in bed thinking about a fight I'd had with Papa when I heard a rock hit my window. I looked out and saw Jerrod's handsome face. He'd come all the way from Big Pine Ranch.

Get dressed, he told me. I pulled on my dress and climbed out the window and down the tree just like a cat. Jerrod helped me up onto his horse and we rode down to the river. It was cold—I know it's going to snow soon because the pine trees are so quiet—and Jerrod gave me his coat. A million stars twinkled overhead. You're different from other girls, Jerrod said to me. You don't let anyone tell you what to do. He touched my face and told me I had beautiful skin. I was gonna say No, it's too dark, but then I decided if he liked my skin, I'd keep my mouth shut. I liked the feel of his hands on me and I didn't want him to stop.

That's when he kissed me. I've always liked kissing boys. But Jerrod's tongue made me feel different. I started to feel wet between my legs. I took his hand and put it there. He said, Are you sure? And I said Hell yes! I could feel him through his pants so I undid them and took him in my hand. He started to groan so I kept doing it. I want you, Earline, he said. I want you too, I told him.

We kissed until I thought I was gonna burst. Then he rolled over on top of me and put his thing inside me. He went really slow but it still hurt. Then it started to feel better. I started to move my hips against him but I'd only been doin that a little while when he let out a big groan and fell down on me. When I got home and back in bed I rubbed myself until I felt like I was joining the stars outside.

I stopped reading the diary and caught my breath. It was one thing to find racy stories in the pages of Victorian erotica; it was another to find true-life erotic confessions in my great-grandmother's diary. But I couldn't put it down.

December 13, 1895. Big blizzard today. Jerrod came here to help Poppa, and then he had to stay the night on account of the snow. I forgot to say what Jerrod looks like. He's not tall but has eyes as blue as Henry's Fork creek, and gold hair like the sun, and a smile that makes my heart beat fast. All night he tried to sneak kisses from me. I told him that Daddy would tan his hide. But then after everyone had gone to sleep, I crept downstairs and crawled under his blanket. He acted like he was shocked but I think he was happy too.

I reached in his longjons and found that he was already hard. I took him in my mouth. Oh my God, Earline, he kept saying, holding on to my long dark hair. Then I climbed up on him so he could taste me. He gobbled at me like I was a turkey but Oh! Did it feel good. But I was too afraid Poppa was gonna hear us so I slid down under the blanket. I rubbed and rubbed myself against him until I felt the lightning shooting through me.

I was overcome by admiration for this woman I'd never known. I had kept a diary once, but I'd put it away when I was thirteen, after my brother narrated a family dinner with an entry about my crush on Billy White. After that, I'd made sure to keep all my feelings about boys hidden—even to them. It had taken Greg months to realize that I liked him as much as he liked me. And here was my Great-Grandma Earline, telling everything!

February 3, 1896. We've had blizzards all winter. I feel like I'm going to jump out of my skin. But today the snow cleared enough for us to make our way into town. Momma talked Poppa into letting us go into town. We were in Mr. Pearson's store when I came around a corner and there was Jerrod. I yelled to Momma and Mr. Pearson that I was gonna get a bag of flour from the back. I dragged Jerrod back to the storeroom. He pushed me up against the wall, hiked up my skirts, and was in me right away. We kept knockin things over and Mr. Pearson hollered at us were we all right. We tried not to laugh. God it's good to see you Earline, Jerrod kept whisperin.

I flipped through the pages. Standard entries about life in late nineteenth-century Wyoming—stories of births, deaths, horses and other gossip—alternated with tales of Earline's erotic adventures. I racked my brain: Was my great-grandfather's name Jerrod? I couldn't remember.

April 3, 1896. I followed Jerrod into the stable and came up behind him as he was saddling Daisy. Why don't you ride me instead, I whispered in his ear. He grinned and kissed me until I felt like I could hardly stand. Then he leaned me back on a haystack so I was on my back and he was standing up. He spread my legs and put himself inside me. I want to touch myself, I told him. Go ahead, he said. So I did and let him watch me.

July 20, 1896. I was out by the creek pickin flowers for Momma's table—bluebells, daisys, Johnny-Jump-ups—when I came round the bend and saw an Indian man lying naked asleep on the bank. His clothes were piled up next to him. His skin was as brown as coffee, and his long shiny black hair was bunched in a pool under his head. He had the most beautiful thing I'd ever seen, thick and red. As I stood there watching him he opened his eyes and raised himself on his elbow. You're not white, he said to me. My dad is, I said. My mom is Shoshone. He nodded. The Snake Tribe, he said.

I'd never seen a man naked in broad daylight and I had to get closer. I slipped out of my dress and lay down next to him. I kissed his neck and his chest and stomach. Then I kissed his thing very gently and it rose up to meet my lips. He turned me onto my hands and knees and put himself into me from

> behind. I'd never done it that way, and I wished I could have looked at him, but I liked how it felt, too. He reached around and rubbed me until I screamed with happiness. Afterwards, we lay together and I held his thing in my hand. I couldn't get enough of it. I told him my name was Earline and he started to laugh. No, I have a name for you. I'm going to call you Red Snake Woman.

Reading the diary, I burst out laughing, too. *Maybe this is why I like sex so much,* I thought to myself. *It's in my blood!* Not that Greg complained about my raging libido, but I felt there was something strange about me. Now I saw how ridiculous that was. Here I was, at the beginning of the twenty-first century, trying to keep my lust in check, while my nineteenth-century great-grandmother seemed to have no qualms about exploring her sexuality to the fullest.

"What's so funny?" a voice asked. I looked up to see Greg standing at the attic door.

"My great-grandmother's diary."

"Is she a comedian?"

"No, she's horny, and not afraid to talk about it."

"Let me see that."

I started to hand it to him, and then I yanked it back. A plan unfurled itself in a corner of my mind. "No. I have a better idea."

That night, as Greg sat at my mother's mahogany dining room table tapping away at his laptop, I crept up behind him and clapped my hands over his eyes. "Close the computer."

"I just have—"

"Close the computer."

He snapped the screen down onto the keyboard, and reached around to touch me. "You're naked!"

"I sure am. Now keep your eyes closed." I dug my fingers into his curly black hair and tilted his head back. I kissed him gently on the lips: once, twice. On the third kiss, I slipped my tongue into his mouth, kissing him at first softly, then deeper. When I stopped, he reached for me, but I pulled away.

"I'll be right back," I said.

I turned off all the lights in the dining room and lit as many candles as I'd been able to find in the cupboards. Then I slipped between Greg and the table and knelt in front of him. He scooted the chair back a few inches to give me room, but he kept his eyes firmly shut. I took my black hair out of its usual ponytail and let it fall around my shoulders.

"You can open your eyes now."

He did, and his eyes took me in.

"Why, Evelyn," he whispered. "Look at you."

I undid his belt and then unbuttoned his fly. To my surprise, his erection pushed against his boxers, and I realized just how long it had been since I'd seduced my lover. He lifted his hips to let me pull his jeans and underwear over his hips. I tossed them aside. Then I leaned forward, running my fingers up his thighs, until I reached his balls and his now nearly erect penis. I gazed at it, imagining it inside me. In our hurried, late-night lovemaking at home, we never took the time to really see or feel each other anymore. Now, it seemed like I was seeing and feeling him all over again.

Never taking my eyes from Greg's face, I took him in my hand and rubbed his hardness against my breasts, even using its tip to tease my nipples. I took the entire length in my mouth so I could wet it with my saliva, and then pulled up so that I just had the tip in my mouth. I started to lick him around the sensitive ridge near the crown while I pumped up and down with my hand. With my other hand, I reached between my legs and stroked myself.

"Jesus, Evie," he moaned.

I stood up and straddled his hips, and then very slowly lowered myself onto him, letting him slip into me a little bit at a time. Putting his hands on my hips, he guided my descent. When, finally, our hips rested together, I began rocking against him, rubbing myself against his pubic bone. The chair creaked under us.

"Think it's going to hold?" Greg whispered.

"It is an antique."

Still inside me, he lifted me and set me on the edge of the heavy dining room table. I heard him push his laptop aside. Then he lowered me to the polished surface as if I were made of the china that lined my grandmother's cabinets. Leaning over me, he began to thrust inside me.

"Have I told you how beautiful you are?" Greg asked, running his hands over my breasts, my nipples, my stomach.

"Not lately."

I clasped my legs around him and reached for his hips. Suddenly, memories of the Thanksgiving dinners I'd had at that table flashed in my mind, and I had an image of my entire family sitting around the table, watching me. But as soon as the thought entered my mind, it was replaced by an image of the beautiful young Earline astride Jerrod's face. *He gobbled at me like I was a turkey but Oh! Did it feel good.*

"Wait!" I said. "I want you to eat me." I couldn't believe how verbal I was being. Usually, I just tried to push his hands or mouth in the right direction and hope he got the idea.

He pulled out of me and started to kneel between my legs.

"Not here," I told him, and led him to the couch in the living room. He lay down, and I climbed on top of him, lowering myself to his mouth. He didn't have to be coaxed. Cradling my bottom in his hands, he teased me until waves of pleasure coursed over my skin.

"I'm getting close, baby," I gasped.

He took one hand off my butt and slowly slipped first one, then two fingers inside my wetness, while teasing my other secret place with his thumb. That was all I could stand. The orgasm shot through my body, arching me backwards.

"I have to feel you inside me," I managed.

I slid down onto his waiting hardness, and with the orgasm still coursing through my body, I pounded against him until he cried out, too.

Afterwards, I lay against his chest, listening to his heart and reveling in the feel of his skin against mine.

"Evie," Greg said.

"Mmmm."

"Marry me."

I felt as though the young Earline was standing in the doorway, watching. I felt her spirit, and the spirit of the man at the river, and the spirit of all my ancestors. Maybe I was imagining things, but I thought I sensed their approval, an approval I'd only sensed in this house.

"I will," I said.

"I don't have a ring yet, but when we get back to Champaign, I'm buying you the most expensive leatherbound journal I can find."

I thought of Red Snake Woman, and smiled.

"Perfect," I said.

TANTRIC EXPERIENCE

Secrets in Your Red-Hot Diary

WOULD YOU LIKE TO LEARN MORE ABOUT HOW YOU achieve your peak sexual experiences? Then write them down! A peak sexual experience can be an earth-moving orgasm, a tender closeness you feel while making love, a oneness with nature while walking in the forest that feels undeniably erotic. Not only are your peak experiences very personal, the way you achieve them is unique to you as well.

You may not know, for example, that you have a tendency to be more turned on—or off—by what you see, what you hear or what you touch (or otherwise sense). Do you think it would be useful to know which of these is your favorite avenue of erotic inspiration?

If you are visual (V), then your appearance and your partner's appearance are very important to you both romantically and sexually. In fact, you would never have been attracted to them in the first place if they did not look good and dress well.

If you are auditory (A), then your partner's voice is the key to your heart. They may be merely okay in the looks department, but if their voice is music to your ears, you don't need much else.

If you are kinesthetic (K), then looks and voice are not as important as how it feels when they touch you. When you get in bed with your mate, the result is always hot, sweet, and sensual.

Complete a Red Hot Diary blank page for each peak sexual experience you want to explore. After working through a few experiences with your diary, you will discover your unique pleasure needs. Knowing what turns you *off* is as important as knowing what turns you *on*!

With the help of your Red Hot Diary, you will know exactly what you want and what you don't want in the bedroom. Self-knowledge is personal power. It is the cornerstone of your tantric pleasure-claiming program. How can you ask for what you want if you don't know what it is?

My Red Hot Diary Page

Season/phase of the moon/my menstrual rhythm:

My mood/stress level:

Description of location:

Sights? Sounds? Touch feelings? Tastes? Smells?

Other environmental elements/distractions:

What my intuition (instincts) sensed:

My expectations (hopes, fears, wishes):

My internal self-talk (sample words/distraction level, 1 to 5):

Personal skill(s) I used:

Tantric/other methods/styles shared:

Did I make erotic sounds?

During lovemaking and orgasm, was I most aware of V, A or K?

My degree of breathing freedom (1 to 5):

My orgasmic satisfaction (1 to 5):

Did I use spoken words effectively?

Did I own my feelings and claim my pleasure (yes or no)?

What did I learn about myself/my partner?

My Red Hot Diary Page
(Sarah's Entries)

Season/phase of the moon/my menstrual rhythm:
Summer. Moon was full. I just finished with my period. No bleeding.

My mood/stress level: *Up mood. Stress low.*

Description of location: *My boyfriend's loft apartment.*

Sights: *Great view of the city lights*

Sounds: *Could hear the traffic below. He put on Steely Dan.*

Touch feelings: *I asked him to give me a neck massage.*

Tastes: *Wine from our trip to Sonoma vineyards last month.*

Smells: *He surprised me with roses—what a sweetie!*

Other environmental elements/distractions: *No, thank god!*

What my intuition (instincts) sensed: *I felt he was really open. I sensed I could take risks, that he was ready for the next level.*

My expectations (hopes, fears, wishes): *I hope it's still special for him to be with me.*

My internal self-talk (sample words/distraction level, 1 to 5): *Distracting self-talk was low (1-2). I said to myself "I hope this dress doesn't make my ass look big. But then I thought about the way he makes love to my breasts."*

Personal skill(s) I used: *I did an appreciation mantra while we were making love. I closed my eyes and said "Thank you! Thank you!"*

Tantric/other methods/styles shared: *We did soul-gazing while drinking wine. He read a poem he wrote for me.*

Did I make erotic sounds? *Yes. This time I didn't care about the neighbors. He said, "Wow, Sarah, you're really enjoying this!"*

During lovemaking and orgasm, was I most aware of V, A or K? *A*

My degree of breathing freedom (1 to 5): *I suddenly realized it was just a 1 or a 2. I was holding my breath. I started to breathe deeply and with him.*

My orgasmic satisfaction (1 to 5): *4. My body was singing!*

Did I use spoken words effectively? *Yes. I asked for a massage.*

Did I own my feelings and claim my pleasure (yes or no)? *Definitely, yes.*

What did I learn about myself/my partner? *I was scared while I did that little dance for him and stripped down to my bra and panties, but he loved it! I learned that bold is good! Also, about my screaming?! He told me that turned him on and made him feel like a great lover. He's more A than I thought. Also, I think the breathing made a difference. I've never breathed so deeply in my life, not during sex, anyway. Not on purpose like that. And breathing together—what a natural high! An amazing night!*

This is the Red Hot Diary page that Sarah from San Francisco submitted at a workshop. We were reviewing past peak experiences in order to learn more from them. I encourage you to use this form to find out what really makes a difference for you whether the positive experience was recent or not. As long as you can remember it, you can learn from it.

It didn't take Sarah long to complete her diary page, yet she learned several valuable sexual secrets: (1) Her partner is more auditory than she thought. (2) It worked to be bold with him, and it felt good to her. (3) She needs to make sounds when she makes love. (4) When she breathes deeply in rhythm with her partner, she feels closer to him. This also creates powerful bonding sounds that appeal to auditory lovers.

Keeping track of your sexual experiences in this way, you will quickly see how to maximize your personal pleasure. You will also gain insight into your partner's needs. Add to your understanding by recording self-pleasure sessions, too.

Enjoy your adventure of self-discovery with your Red Hot Diary. Have fun with it! Use playful supplies like crayons, markers, paint, glued objects, and pictures. Draw mandalas. Write poetry. Compose a love letter to yourself or your partner. Check Red Hot Resources (at the back of this book) for more journaling resources.

In the story, Evelyn and Greg gain inspiration from the diary of Evelyn's nineteenth-century great-grandmother. Earline Runningwater Stewart loved making love. Her sex-positive attitude and rich, sensual enjoyment awaken Evelyn to a passionate truth: Don't delay! Make love today! It's beautiful!

Compared to the good old days of the Wild West, you have extraordinary technological distractions and a busy, demanding schedule. Today, like it or not, you need to schedule some love-making in just like everything else. What you lack in Wild West spontaneity, you can make up by taking advantage of modern benefits like red-hot tantra techniques, the many varieties of vibrators, sex toys, and games, and fast transportation to a local getaway or exotic distant locales for a totally tantric escape.

TANTRIC TALE

Rain

DURING THE VERY HEIGHT OF THE RAINY SEASON, TOM AND Julie make love every night for twenty days straight. On the weekends, they even do it two or three times a day. For Tom, it begins to become a habit, like brushing his teeth or shaving, albeit a much more pleasurable one.

In truth, there's not much else to do, because the rain has turned their front yard into a swamp and their backyard into a rain forest. The streets have become rivers that flow and break around the wheels of parked cars. It doesn't even seem worth the effort to go downtown. Every time they get out of the car, the rain decides to come at them sideways, soaking their clothes. After a while, they only leave the house to go to work and the grocery store.

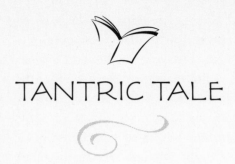

At night they cook themselves elaborate meals to the sound of the rain, challenging each other to see who can find the most exotic recipe. Salad of poached red trout, Belgian endive, and watercress. Pomegranate soup. Roast pheasant with forty cloves of garlic. They don't even bother to put a CD on the stereo. They cook in happy silence, their only accompaniment the sound of knives on cutting boards, the crack and sizzle of food hitting a hot pan, and, as always, the drum of rain on the roof. Then they turn off the lights, and eat to the light of the fireplace and candles.

Sometimes they eat without talking, gazing at each other over the table. Tom can't take his eyes off Julie, and the way her red curly hair catches the light. Her eyes, when she looks at him from above her wine glass, are as green as the ferns that, after two weeks of steady rainfall, threaten to consume their garden. It takes him superhuman effort to keep himself from pushing the plates aside and going at it right there on the dining room table, but they found on Night Two of the deluge that full stomachs and fucking don't mix.

So he waits until they've cleared the table and washed the dishes. Tom waits until the moment when she turns to him, every night, presses herself against him, and asks innocently, "What do you want to do now?"

Usually, they don't even make it to the bedroom. He'll start kissing her, she'll wrap her legs around him, and before they know it they're on the couch, the deep blue couch that's like a raft on a stormy sea. He pulls off her sweatpants and throws them to the floor; he yanks off her T-shirt and lobs it into the dining room. She does the same to his shorts and shirt. She lies on top of him and wraps her full lips around his erection while he lifts his head, tongue first, into her sweet garden. Then they make love: Sometimes she's on top; sometimes he is. Sometimes she sits back against the cushion as he kneels in front of her. Sometimes he's behind her as they watch the rain come down in sheets. They try every position in the Kama Sutra, and then make up some of their own. He imagines that when he comes, the rain gets louder.

And then, after twenty days, the rain stops.

There's no warning: They wake up one morning, and the sun is shining. In honor of the nice weather, Tom decides that they should have a picnic, and he buys a baguette, duck pâté, and Havarti cheese from the corner deli. She opens a bottle of Chardonnay, he puts a Bach CD on the stereo, and they eat side by side on teak chairs in the backyard.

"The sun feels good," he says as he spreads pâté onto a piece of bread.

"It sure does," she says.

After dinner, she presses against him as usual. "What do you want to do now?" she says.

He kisses her in the kitchen. He kisses her in the living room. Finally, they go to the bedroom, and he kisses her there.

He can't get hard.

Julie pushes him back on the pillows. She kneels between his legs and kisses the tip of his penis. She licks it like a lollipop. She pours lube into her palms and strokes him until he can see the muscles in her arms straining. His recalcitrant member just lies there, stubbornly flaccid.

"It's not you," he tells her.

He can tell she doesn't believe him, so he rolls her onto her back and sets to work on her, licking and nuzzling and sucking her until she comes with great loud cries that send the cat bolting from the room. Often her excitement is enough to get him going, but not this time. It's as if his penis is saying, *You can eat her until your tongue falls off. I'm not getting up for anyone, dude.*

After the third day, measures are taken. Books consulted. Herbal remedies consumed. Massages given. Nothing works. Meanwhile, in the backyard, roses begin to peek out from their buds. Hummingbirds zip to and fro, taunting Tom with their sharp, long, hard beaks. Tulip bulbs poke up from the ground.

"How come Nature can get a hard-on, but I can't?" he asks her. He stares at the flowering of their garden.

"Maybe we should take a sex break," she suggests. "Give the little man time to recover."

After a week, they begin eating dinner in front of the TV.

"American peasants," he jokes, but she doesn't laugh.

The next day when Tom comes home from work, Julie isn't there. He walks into the bedroom and sees a note folded on his pillow. *That's it,* he thinks. *She's left me.* But the note simply says to make himself comfortable until she gets back.

He sits on the couch and tries to read a book, but his eyes keep darting to the clock.

Finally, at 8:30, he hears her car in the driveway. She comes in the front door with a smile on her face. In one hand she holds a shopping bag from a gourmet food store; the other hand holds a bag she hides behind her back.

"Go take a shower," she says. "A long one. Don't ask questions."

He obeys her. He stands under the showerhead until his skin begins to wrinkle.

When he comes out, he glances down the hallway and sees that the curtains are drawn and the house is dark except for a fire in the fireplace and the glow of several candles scattered around the living room. He smells garlic, onions. His stomach rumbles.

"What are you doing in there?" he calls. "I'm starving."

"Go into the bedroom and lie down."

He puts on a pair of boxer shorts, stretches out on the bedspread and closes his eyes. Suddenly she is there beside him, pulling him into a sitting position. She ties a silk scarf around his eyes and leads him to the dining room. She sits him down on the couch.

"What's this all about?" he asks.

"Shhhh. Listen."

Then he hears it. Quietly, at first. Then louder.

Rain. In the room with them.

He shakes his head. There hasn't been a cloud in the sky for days. "Is it ... how can it be ... raining?"

"Yes," she whispers in his ear. "What do you want to do now?"

He doesn't have to answer. His erection has parted the opening in his shorts and is straining toward the ceiling. He grabs it and strokes it madly, welcoming it back to life. He feels like the rain is everywhere, an insistent drumbeat in his head that mimics the pulsing of his nerves.

"Dinner will have to wait," she says. She pushes his hand aside and takes him in her mouth.

A short time later, he is thrusting into Julie when the scarf falls away from his eyes, and he sees the rain. Or, more accurately, he sees what's making the rain: a brand-new sound machine in the corner, next to the stereo. It's top-of-the-line. It's a boulder of electronic sound excellence. It must have cost her a fortune.

She sees him see it. "It's got settings for the ocean. A babbling brook. An Amazon rain forest."

"I like the rain."

She giggles. "Me too."

He stares at her fern-green eyes and the coppery river of her hair, and kisses her. Then he closes his eyes again, and hears the rain, and comes.

TANTRIC EXPERIENCE

Secret Sensuality of Sound

HAVE YOU EXPERIENCED THE PURE PHYSICALITY, THE SECRET sensuality of sound?

Your whole body can listen, all at once. Then it is ready to become one with the universe. The universe is always making love with the body, always touching it, always caressing it with streams and rivers and bursts of energy and sound. This is the music of life. The body and the universe are always dancing to it.

The body does not know that it is separate from its environment. In fact, it is not. Were it not for the fact of this oneness, the senses could not operate. No connection could be made.

You think you are separate, and you think your body is separate. But it is not, and you are not. It is so only in your thinking. But thinking does not make it so. Thinking only makes more thinking!

Be the body only. Be the body in its wholeness. Discover its oneness with space, with its surroundings. Listen to the silence, to the emptiness of the sounds coming from the space that expands from the body in every direction. Sense this nourishing space.

It surrounds the body. It touches, kisses, caresses, loves, and feeds the body.

Attentive in this way, there is no mind—there is only listening. It is not you that listens. The body is always already listening. In that natural listening, there is the silent surrender. Listening as the whole body, there is only this listening, only being.

The sounds, the silence, they were there all the time.

Only you did not hear them.

Sound is physical—it is sound waves. These waves are like ocean waves. You live in a sea of sound. Sound is all around you. Right now. Listen. The eardrum is physical—it really is a drum.

Sound waves are touching, tapping, playing it now. The sea of sound is lapping in waves at your ear. Can you hear this intimate sea? Can you hear the intimacy? Listen with your whole body. Lay on your back. Feel your back against the floor, on the ground.

Become your back, and feel the contact. Feel how the ground touches your back. Become the sense of touch that is your skin. Notice that this touch sensitivity is in your skin everywhere, at every point. Notice that this sense of touch is all over your body.

Now notice the space that surrounds your body, where this sensitivity to touching that is the essence of your skin meets space. This space is awakened by your whole body listening all at once. Listen, now, with the space that surrounds your body. It is already there. You do not have to create it. Just listen. Listen with your whole body. Listen with the space around your body. Listen with your whole body, all at once, from this space.

Feel your skin. Listen with your skin and the space around your skin.

As you feel with your skin, and sense sound with the space around your skin, include your spine in this awareness. Be in your spine, your very alive, electromagnetic, subtly singing spine, as you feel and listen with your whole body all at once.

Be in your spine and move your attention *up* your spine.
Be in your spine and move your attention *down* your spine.
Be in your spine and move your attention *up* your spine.
Be in your spine and move your attention *down* your spine.

Be in your spine and move your attention *up* your spine.

Be in your spine and move your attention *down* your spine.

Now, just let go. Just relax. Float. Let go. Be. Just be. Just be. Just be. Just be.

You have just used listening to enter into the spaciousness of pure Being. Pure Being is the ground of tantra, the heart of space, the essence of orgasm, the majesty of nature, the sound of silence. You are That.

This is wonderful just before going to sleep. It's also very good preparation for making love, or listening to healing music, or meditation.

It reduces stress. It pampers you into the nourishing now. It takes you on a gentle, invisible journey to your spiritual home to nest, rest, relax, and renew in the boundless generosity of silence. This technique for getting in touch with skin, sound, and spine, as one, is yoga knowledge many thousands of years old.

Om Shanti, Shanti, Shanti.

Om Peace, Peace, Peace.

Om. Om. Om.

Ommmmmmmmmmmmmmmmmmmmmmmmmm.

In our culture, we tend to relegate sound and music to the background—in the elevator, in the car, as the soundtrack for movies or television. When you make love, though, sound is second only to sight. When you close your eyes, sound moves forward and takes the driver's seat.

Is there anything sexier than the sounds your lover makes when you give them pleasure? Close your eyes and listen to the closeness. It is caressing your living, loving skin all at once through your eardrums. Awakening your skin as a whole, the sensual sounds are touching your soul.

In the story, Tom and Julie celebrate the sweet, sexy secret of sound. That Tom could not get it up without hearing the rain is closer to the truth than you may think. Often there are cues and clues that our brain requires for heightened erotic response. You may know what they are—or you may not.

By playing with all the senses, by actively making sounds and actively listening, you will hear for yourself the difference that sound can make when you make beautiful music together. Just as Julie realized Tom's need before he did, enjoying and exploring the smorgasbord of sound possibilities with each other is a great way to get together and stay together.

TANTRIC TALE

Biker Bar Babe

I walk into the Wagon Wheel, trying to ignore the leers of the leather-clad men leaning against the wall outside. I tug at the waistband of my low-slung jeans, but it's no use: They barely cover the top of my thong panties. What was I thinking? I shake off my leather jacket. Catching sight of my cleavage in a mirror, I start to fasten another button on the red gingham blouse I'm wearing. Then I realize that it's too late for modesty. My entire stomach is already on display, because earlier, I made the questionable decision to tie my shirt up under my breasts. *I must look like an escapee from a porno version of "The Beverly Hillbillies,"* I think. The idea makes me smile, and I get a second wind of confidence. I saunter up to the bar as best I can on four-inch spiked-heeled boots.

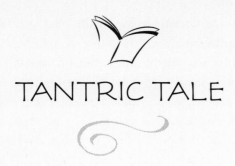

I catch myself before I order my usual Cosmo. I'm in a biker bar, for God's sake. So I get a bottle of Bud, perch on a bar stool, and survey my surroundings. For a dive, it's not such a bad place. With its red brocade wallpaper, torn naugahyde booths, and Harley Davidson insignia behind the bar, the décor has seen better days, but at least the place has character. I give the dot-com refugees another year to discover and ruin it.

I've just begun to relax when I notice several men at the bar staring at me. I cross my legs, and my thong immediately rides all the way up my crack. It's all I can do not to reach my hand into the back of my pants and give it a good yank. Instead, I sit up straight and pretend that I'm just trying to rearrange the back of my jeans. Big mistake. At the end of the bar, a large, hairy man with a gray ponytail and pockmarked face grins at me. My subtle rearrangements, it seems, have come across as lust-induced squirming. Another thirty seconds and he'll be heading my way. Shit.

Just in time, you walk in and sidle up next to Mr. Ponytail, distracting him. My heart jumps—in relief or excitement, I'm not sure. I look at you almost as a stranger might, as if I haven't been looking at you every day for two years. In your tight black leather pants and heavy black leather jacket, your dark hair close-cropped to your scalp, your full mouth unsmiling, you look remote and dangerous, just like the first time I saw you. It's perfect. You nod to Mr. Ponytail, and I admire the strong hook of your nose.

Your dark eyes catch mine. Normally if I were in this kind of situation, I would feign interest in the lettering of my beer label. Instead, I narrow my eyes and stare back at you. The strength of our gaze creates a cord of lust between us. Mr. Ponytail looks first at you, then at me, amazed.

After a beat or two, you amble slowly over to me. The musky oiliness of your leathers fills my nose. I want to touch you. Not yet, I tell myself. You order two tequila shots, put one in front of me and lean close, so that there's only an inch between us. I can feel your breath on my cheek.

"Hey, Dorothy. Where's Toto?" Your voice is deep, raspy, sarcastic.

I want to laugh, but when I glance at you, I see that you aren't smiling. Wow, I think. You're really getting into this. I decide that I will, too. After all, it was my idea. I look you straight in the eye.

"Probably out screwing some bitch," I say. I feel a surge of power.

"Wish I were doing the same."

"Who knows? If you stop yapping, maybe you'll get lucky." Another surge.

In answer, you take the back of an index finger and run it up the inside of my thigh, stopping just at the top. It's as though you've touched me with a live electric wire: I'm wet instantly. I push your hand away firmly and look you up and down, pausing significantly at your crotch.

"So you got anything else going for you other than that big hog?" I purr.

"You mean the one parked outside?"

I pause. "Yeah. The one parked outside."

"Let me take you for a ride."

"I wouldn't mind a spin on your motorcycle, either," I say, not taking my eyes off the bulge in your pants. I can't believe the words have come out of my mouth—and I'm surprised at how good they feel. *God, it's fun to be bad*, I think.

"Don't know about that. It's pretty big. Can you handle it?"

"I've ridden some big hogs in my day."

"I'll bet."

You slap a twenty onto the bar. We throw back our shots, and without another word, I head for the door. I emphasize every step so you can enjoy the sway of my ass. I can feel eyes on me, and I imagine what Mr. Ponytail is thinking. If only he knew!

The cold night air hits my bare stomach as we step outside. You hand me a helmet, because as much as we're enjoying this little fantasy game, neither of us is going to throw caution to the wind. I gaze at your gleaming Harley.

"Nice," I say. "I can hardly wait to feel it between my legs."

You don't even break a smile. "Where do you live?"

I pause, as though I'm considering whether to give you my address, and then tell you. You nod. You mount the bike, and motion me toward the back with a nod of your head. "Get on," you say roughly.

I lower the helmet visor, put on my gloves, and straddle the cushion. I press myself against your back, tilting my hips ever so slightly. When you start the engine and put the bike into gear, I'm rewarded: The motor sends a rough vibration directly between my legs. My entire body begins to quiver, as though I've mounted a giant vibrator. As we speed down the street, I remember again why I like your motorcycle so much. There's nothing between me and the outside world. There's nothing protecting me. Nothing except you.

Luckily, we don't have far to go.

I walk slowly in front of you up the two flights of stairs to the apartment. I want to make sure you get a good look at my ass, because I know how much you like it. As we reach the second flight, you push me against the wall, shoving your crotch into mine. With one hand you grope my breasts, the other my butt, and you shove your tongue into my mouth.

"Simmer down, dude," I say when I come up for air.

"I want you."

"You'll get me."

You continue to grope and fondle me as I struggle with my keys at the door, but inside the apartment, I pull away. I light candles, put Faith Hill on the CD player and turn it up loud. I open a couple of beers. You don't say a word. You just watch me.

"Dance with me," I say, taking your hands in mine. We two-step for a few beats, and then you pull me close.

"Dancing's for pussies. Let's get to the action."

We crush our mouths together. Our tongues lash at each other. I slide my hand up your shirt and rake my nails down your back. I stick my hand down the back of your pants, taking a handful of your delicious, firm butt. You reciprocate by grabbing my ass, lifting me off the floor, and carrying me to the dining room table, where you set me down with a thud.

We can't get our clothes off fast enough. You pull off my boots, then my jeans. I yank your shirt over your head. You hook a finger into the thin strip of fabric that passes for my underwear and push them to one side. I'm so wet that when you put your middle finger inside me, it slips in easily. You raise an eyebrow.

"You're wet."

"Horny for you."

You move the finger in and out while you massage my clitoris with your thumb. With your other hand you untie my shirt and rip it open—it's from the thrift store, so I don't really care—sending the buttons ricocheting against the wall. You push my bra up over my breasts and suck at my nipples.

By this time, all I know is that I have to have you inside me. I reach for your belt buckle, but you push my hands away.

"Stop it," you growl, pushing me back onto the table. "Play with your tits."

I wrap my legs around you and comply, rubbing my nipples back and forth between my fingers as you pump away with your finger, your thumb still against me, matching the rhythm of my fingers, starting up a vibration way more intense than the motorcycle. I buck against your fingers like a wild pony. With your other hand you undo your fly and release your gorgeous erection—you're not wearing underwear—from the confines of your tight pants.

"Stroke yourself," I order you. "Get yourself ready for me."

I look at your penis—large, dark, rock-hard—and imagine it inside me. I let go of what usually holds me back. What does it matter? Right now, I can be as wild as I want. You press harder on me. Without warning, I feel myself on the edge of orgasm. I can't believe it. I never come this fast.

"Oh my God," I gasp. "I think I'm going to come."

"Do it," you order me.

And I do, hard, as though your finger inside me is injecting me with an orgasm that shoots like lit gasoline through my veins, sparks flying down my nerve endings. I feel like I could come forever. Just before I become too sensitive, you pull your fingers away, plunge yourself into me, and grab my hips, slamming into me like a piston. All I can feel are your thrusts. You're like a machine, banging up against my womb. Finally, my orgasm subsides, and I sit up and pull your mouth to mine. You let me kiss you, but you don't stop your thrusts. I lie back on the cold wood of the table and arch my back so that I can feel you against me. I know you're getting close. I rock my hips a little in the way I know you like, and I watch as your face twists and strains. You come, yelling out, and collapse into me.

It takes us several minutes to recover. "Wow," you say into my neck. "I think I like picking you up in biker bars."

"Didn't know you had such a tough guy in you, did you?"

"Nah. Didn't know you did, either."

"I still do," I answer, squirming my hips to feel you still hard inside me.

Laughing, you lift me up, and carry me to the couch. We fall onto it, and you pull a blanket over us. Finally, I feel you slide out of me. I miss you immediately.

"God, that was fun," I say. And it was. I remember how much I loved playing make-believe games when I was a kid. Tonight recaptured that feeling. I feel re-energized, as though I could stay up all night.

"So what's next?" you ask. "You wouldn't happen to have any streetwalker fantasies, would you?"

Laughing, I kiss you. The idea is tantalizing. But I have a feeling that tonight has resolved something in me. I won't need to be a biker bar babe, or anyone else, for a long time. I won't need to be anyone else except me. But for now, I reach for you again. The biker bar babe, it seems, isn't quite ready to go to sleep.

TANTRIC EXPERIENCE

Tantric Role-Playing

HERE IS MY SPECIAL APPROACH TO TANTRIC ROLE-PLAYING. It draws upon classical tantric imagery of god and goddess, yet inspires playfulness, even wonder.

To do my "Play God/Goddess for a Day" technique, you do not need to be lovers. In my workshops, people pair off who have never met before. In truth, this technique helps reveals the divine within, which transcends all roles, races, and sexual preferences.

One person chooses to be the devotee. The other is the god (male personage) or goddess (female personage). After you complete the experience, then you will switch roles. The devotee becomes the deity, and vice versa.

Begin by sitting across from each other. If you are playing the god or goddess, say nothing. Only smile. At the very end, when the devotee is finished praising you, you will say a few words and bless them.

In an easy and effortless way, the god or goddess does what he or she can to generate unconditional love and send it to the devotee.

However, great ease, great contentment, great peace is the mood of the deity. So, just relax and enjoy!

If you are playing the devotee in this experience, you will do most of the work. After a few minutes of meditation with eyes closed, you speak. You praise the deity and glorify them. I will give you a verbal formula you can follow, if you like.

You begin the simple, eyes-closed meditation. Visualize the other as a god or goddess with a third eye in their forehead and a tangible glow around their body. Also see them in your mind's eye as physically very beautiful or handsome.

If you like, you can imagine jeweled ornaments, such as diamond rings, emerald bracelets, a ruby necklace touching their flawless skin, a crown or tiara encrusted with many gems resting upon their perfect body. Finally, encourage a special devotional feeling. In words, this special mood might say "I am in the presence of a sacred being."

This is the first step. Now comes the best part, which makes "Play God/Goddess for a Day" as powerful as it is playful. Now you speak out loud to your deity what you have visualized in your mind's eye.

Deity and devotee look at each other. They gently hold each other's gaze. This is a unique, sacred, precious moment. It is not often that you get to meet a real god or goddess, or that you get to be one!

"Oh, great goddess, you have a beautiful violet third eye in your forehead. This is incredible, but I can see it. And your body is entirely surrounded by a bright, beautiful golden glow. You are beautiful beyond words. Your ornaments are those of a queen. From you emanate and radiate lovely, sweet, amazing vibrations of perfect love, bliss, and peace. Truly, I am overwhelmed. I feel so unworthy, so undeserving. Please grace me with your blessings. I am made speechless."

You don't need to say these exact words. The "secret" is that you speak out loud these deifying visualizations so that the person playing the god or goddess can hear them, feel them, and see themselves with those divine attributes.

You, as the devotee, are invoking the inner deity of the human god or goddess in front of you. You are inviting the divine within them to come out, to be present. You have asked them to share it with you. They will feel it. When you are done praising them, sit once again briefly in silence. This time sit with eyes open. Look at each other.

When the time is right, the god or goddess replies. "You are my beloved devotee, in whom I am well pleased. Know that you are perfect. Know that you are totally and unconditionally loved. Behold, I am with you always. I bestow upon you my blessings and my grace. May you fully realize your inner divine nature. May you be one with the supreme self that lives in the hearts of all beings. That I am. That you are."

Again, the exact words are not important. The spirit, the feeling, the sincerity of your words, be they few or many, is the key. Zen-like gruff or poetically rolling, down-to-earth simple or flagrantly flowery, it doesn't matter. Just speak from your heart.

When the deity is done speaking, and the fullness of the moment has passed, give each other a hug. In workshops, I have heard both laughter and crying during this exercise. But the tears are always of joy, the joy of tasting your intrinsic divinity.

This experience draws upon the imagery of gods and goddesses from the Hindu and Buddhist tantric traditions. Look at their beautiful artwork for inspiration and ideas.

Somehow, to imagine that you or another person has a wide-open, physical third eye in the forehead and a brightly glowing aura surrounding the body causes a change in consciousness. It triggers a worshipful mood, a sense of awe, a spirit of wonder. This visualization is the key element. I have watched it work its magic at many workshops.

Self-liberating role-play can recharge a flagging relationship and juice up a boring sex life. Other rewards include deeper empathy and rapport with each other, psychological empowerment and the discovery of new talents, skills, and turn-ons.

You will probably find this principle of acting "as if" introduces you to delightful new ways to interact with each other. You will discover new inner treasures that deepen shared pleasures, bringing the two of you closer together than ever before.

Through conscious role-playing, you can also access the power of your shadows together, enriching your connection with its dark soil. The gold you cannot see is hidden in the shadow you do not know. For more on how to work with your erotic shadow selves, see the sections "Truth Through Fantasy" and "Tantric S&M."

A little tantric role-play goes a long way. You are accessing, energizing, and taking into your life great universal, eternal archetypes. When you plug your intimacy into cosmic sources, the sky is the limit!

In the story, a sophisticated couple digs deep and discovers the power of fulfilling each other's raw, outlaw fantasies. By unleashing their private lust in a public setting, they find they can be the other lover with each other. They can have it all, do it all, be it all—and still have each other!

Uninhibited role-playing helps strengthen their relationship. Sometimes the best way to solidify your connection is the baddest!

TANTRIC TALE

Tantric Slut Guru

If you saw me downtown, you'd think I was any other young professional woman. You'd be right. I do have a profession: I am a slut. A tart, bawd, harlot, courtesan, prostitute. A call girl with an exclusive clientele, a closet full of designer clothes, an upper West Side loft, and a tax accountant. A whore with a bachelor's degree in psychology from Columbia, and a master's degree in anthropology from Harvard. A slut with a calling.

Because it is a calling to me. Like the sacred temple prostitutes of ancient Babylonia, I offer men—and occasionally, women—a service that, more times than you'd think, doesn't even involve sex, but always involves their souls. I am a guru of spiritual sex. A tantric slut guru.

But a tantric slut guru whose days are drawing to a close.

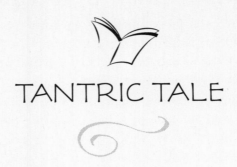

A regular client referred Jack to me. I ran the usual background check and credit report, and had him fill out my online questionnaire. Jack was squeaky clean. He'd made a bundle out in Silicon Valley during the dot-com boom and had had the sense—or the luck—to cash out before the crash. Now he occupied his time with building a house in San Francisco. *I love being outdoors,* he said in the questionnaire, adding that he was training for a triathlon. He doesn't love nature, I thought. He loves his body. He went on to describe himself as a "serial monogamist." I doubted that, too.

In my five years in business, I've found something to like in every client, but I found myself ready to hate Jack. I pictured an arrogant asshole in a BMW, a sheltered jerk with no idea of the real world and an overdeveloped idea of his own invincibility. I resigned myself to several hours of loving-kindness meditation and prepared for him like I'd prepare for any other client, brushing up on high tech and San Francisco real estate prices. Then I went to the studio I rent in the Village for my sessions. My temple.

Given Jack's supposed love of the outdoors, I went with a Camping in the Village theme for my temple that night. I replaced the red velvet canopy around the bed with white linen curtains as thin as mosquito netting, put clean, white sheets on the bed, and bought pine-scented candles. In the living room, I spread a large blanket in front of the fireplace and surrounded it with cushions. I dressed in a red sports bra to show off my abs and breasts, and low-slung khaki pants. I pulled my long blonde hair into a high ponytail and kept my makeup to a minimum. The Rock-Climbing Slut Next Door.

I meditated for an hour to release the negative image of Jack I'd built up in my mind. I visualized this image floating away, like a twig on a forest stream.

Jack was on time. That was my first surprise. The more money someone has, the more cavalier they usually are about other people's time, even if they're paying for it. My second surprise came when I opened the door.

At one time, Jack must have been a good-looking guy. He was about 5'10",with wavy, dark-blonde hair cut very short; a strong nose; a smile that revealed strong, white perfect teeth; and a dimpled chin. I could tell, even under his crew-neck shirt and jeans, that he didn't have an ounce of fat on him. But it was his blue eyes that really surprised me. It was his eyes that kept him from being handsome.

I've met a lot of stressed-out, worn-out men, but until that moment, I'd never seen a man, especially one of his age, whose eyes were so dead. It was as though every ounce of life had been drained out of them. He looked, standing there with his hands in his pockets, like an exhausted angel. I reached out my arms, and enfolded him.

"Welcome, Jack," I whispered. "I'm Alison."

I led him to the blanket, told him to take off his shoes, and went to the refrigerator for a couple of beers. He sat on the edge of the blanket as if he were ready to bolt, watching me like a scared deer. When I handed him his bottle and our fingers touched, he almost jumped. *He hasn't touched a woman in a while,* I thought.

He took a long swig. "I've never done this before."

"Don't worry. 'This' can be whatever you want. It's your night."

He brightened, and for a moment, I saw a flash of life. "I don't know where to start," he said. "Do I touch you, or . . ."

"You can if you want. But first just tell me why you're in New York." I leaned back on a cushion and stretched out my legs.

"To see friends. I wanted to take a break from the Bay Area."

"From *someone* in the Bay Area."

His blue eyes widened. "How did you know that?"

"I guessed." It hadn't been hard. Defeat clung to him like a wet shirt, but it wasn't the kind of defeat born of a lost deal or job setback. Defeat in areas of the heart always has its own stale aroma. "We can talk about it if you want. But we don't have to."

He stared at his bottle for a long time before he spoke. "She said I wasn't ambitious enough. That I wasn't sexy enough."

I found that hard to believe and told him so. I asked him questions and let him talk, never taking my eyes from his face. Slowly, he began to confide in me about his ex-girlfriend. He hadn't seen the breakup coming; as his new house had taken shape, he'd imagined her in it, their children running up and down the hallways. I listened and nodded. It wasn't losing the person that was so hard. It was the dream, the illusion.

He slumped against the cushions. "And since then, I've been going on these nightmare blind dates. I just can't seem to connect with anyone."

How can you give to anyone if you don't have anything left to give? I thought. I paused, then reached for him. "Come here."

I took him in my arms, held him for a while, and slowly, gently, began to kiss his hair and face as I rocked him. I could feel the tension leaving his body.

"I want to kiss you," he said suddenly.

I was surprised, but pleased. "Good. I really want to feel your tongue in my mouth."

Without hesitation, Jack turned his lips to mine. As we kissed, I could feel the hunger in his mouth and tongue. "You're a great kisser," I said when we finally paused.

I sat up and pulled his shirt over his head. He definitely had a triathlete's body. I ran my hands over his strong chest and his smooth, defined abs. While I appreciated his beauty, I wouldn't have cared if he'd had a beer belly and tits bigger than mine. Some of my most sensitive, passionate clients—and my most skilled lovers—have been guys that other girls would reject. It's the gorgeous guys who are often the most inept in bed, and that's what I expected from Jack. I leaned him back on the cushions and teased his nipples with my tongue.

"What do you like to do in bed, Jack?" I said.

"My girlfriend never liked to talk dirty," he replied in a whisper.

"Do you mind if I talk dirty now?"

"No." His voice was both nervous and excited.

"Because I think I'd like to suck you. Then I want you to fuck me."

"That sounds good." His voice was almost inaudible.

I reached down, unbuttoned his jeans and pulled them off. His erection sprang from the opening in his boxer shorts. I leaned my head to its tip and kissed it, teasing it with my tongue. A quiet moan came from Jack's lips. I eased his boxers over his hips.

"I want to see you naked," he said. The flicker in his eyes grew brighter.

I stood and undressed, as his eyes devoured my body from the top of my head to my pubic hair, down my legs to the tips of my toes. As he watched me, I felt a strange sensation, as though I were naked in front of a man for the first time. What I felt from him was more than mere appreciation or lust. Then I understood: in his own way, Jack was worshipping me. My face grew warm.

I quickly knelt between his legs, and took his penis in one hand and his balls in another. I paused, gazing at it as reverently as if it were an ivory phallus in a temple, a religious icon. It seemed to grow harder under my eyes.

"Do you like it?" he asked shyly. I could tell from his tone that his girlfriend had probably never really looked at it.

"I love it. It's beautiful. I want to suck it. I want to suck it bad."

I bent down and again began sucking the tip, slowly taking more and more of it into my mouth as I continued to stroke it with one hand, so that I was giving him both a hand job and a blow job. Meanwhile, I gently caressed his balls.

"Oh my God, that feels amazing," he whispered. "I … I really want to eat you."

Again, I was surprised: I hadn't expected him to be the kind of guy who likes to give a woman pleasure. I swiveled around and straddled his face, never taking my mouth from his erection. I felt him reach out a hand and stroke my ass. It was the first time he'd touched my naked skin, and it tingled where his fingers made contact. He pulled my hips down to his mouth. I felt him kiss my lower lips, then part them with his tongue and gently lick me. I moaned, but I wasn't faking. Usually, until I show men what to do, their tongues flap away like they were licking envelopes. But Jack knew what he was doing,

"God, you eat me good," I moaned. "You eat me *so* good. Lick my clit. Lick it hard."

He didn't need any encouragement. His tongue was like a finger, flicking the hard button back and forth insistently. I caught myself before I gave in to the pleasure. I needed to right the balance. I pivoted around back between his knees.

"Wait, I want to keep eating you," he protested.

"Later. First, I want to ride this beautiful thing."

I pulled out a condom from under the cushions, and unrolled it onto him. I straddled him, and I touched his hardness to my already wet entrance.

"Do you want to fuck me, Jack?"

"Yeah, I want to fuck you. I want to fuck you hard."

"What? I can't hear you. And I'm not gonna give you this until I can hear you."

"I want to fuck you," he said, louder.

I let him slip into me an inch. I tightened my muscles around him and narrowed my eyes. "What? Is this what you want? Speak up, Jack. Speak up if you want to fuck me."

He drew his breath in. "Yeah. I want to fuck you."

It became like a call and response. Every time he told me he wanted to fuck me, I made him repeat himself, and when he did, I slid down onto him another inch. If he didn't say it loud enough, I pulled up until he shouted his desire. Finally, he was completely inside me. I began to move on top of him slowly, building speed. Never did I take my eyes from his, and in truth, I wouldn't have wanted to miss the change coming over him. It was as though someone were turning up a dimmer switch behind his pupils. He ran his hands up my hips to my breasts and tweaked my nipples until they were hard.

"God, I love it when you rub my tits while you're fucking me," I moaned. "You feel so good. Fuck me. Fuck me, Jack. Fuck me hard."

By this time, Jack didn't need my encouragement. "I'll fuck you. Yeah, I'll fuck you hard. You like that, don't you? You like me fucking you. You like me inside you."

He clutched my hips and ground me to his pelvis as I bounced on him. I hardly recognized him as the sallow-faced man who'd come through my door an hour before. His skin glowed with a fine sheen of perspiration; his cheeks flushed with excitement. Best of all, he was smiling. Jack was having fun with a woman for the first time in a long while.

I saw the muscles in his stomach and jaws began to stiffen and knew that he was approaching orgasm. I slowed my movements. "I want you on top of me," I growled.

He quickly rolled me over onto my back. His thrusts were long, deep, hard. He began swiveling his hips so that he reached parts of me I didn't know existed. I screamed in honest delight and wrapped my legs around his back. Grabbing his butt, I pulled him into me.

"Yes, Jack. Screw me just like that. Just like that! Like that! Oh my God. You're a fucking sex machine. A fucking, non-stop sex machine." Porn-movie dialogue, I know, but it worked. Jack pounded into me.

"I want to come inside you. I want to shoot inside you."

"Yes! Do it! Do it, Jack!"

Suddenly, with a growl that came from somewhere deep in his chest, Jack began to come. He arched up away from me, his eyes widening in surprise as the orgasm took over, the flush suffusing his chest and face. Finally, he collapsed against my breasts, panting. I stroked his back from the cleft of his buttocks to the top of his shoulders, spreading the afterglow across his skin. His breathing slowed, and for a moment, I thought he had fallen asleep. Then he nuzzled my breast.

"Thank you," he whispered. "That was amazing."

"You're welcome."

"Did you enjoy it at all?" He paused, shook his head. "I can't believe I just asked you that."

I took his chin and raised his face so that he could look at me. I saw that his eyes had come back to life, but I knew that with a word, I could extinguish the flame. "You really, really are a wonderful lover." It was true, and inside I grieved a little to think that he thought it wasn't.

He grinned.

"*Now* you're supposed to say, 'Thank you,'" I said.

He laughed. "Thank you."

"You're welcome. Now let's have something to eat."

Jack and I snacked and talked for hours. The next time we had sex, we talked dirty again, but the third time, we made love in silence on my white bed, the curtains drawn around us as though we were deep in some primeval jungle. This time, as he moved inside me, I told him to just let himself feel.

I never let my clients spend the night, but at some point, Jack and I fell asleep on the bed, our bodies intertwined, and when I woke up, the sky was just beginning to lighten. I kissed him awake.

"Jack, wake up. You have to go."

I watched him slowly remember where he was.

"Oh my God. I'm sorry. Do I . . . owe you more?"

My disappointment caught me by surprise, and through the disappointment, a voice spoke as clear as a church bell: *You've just had your last client.* I was so stunned that I kept my back to him as I got out of bed and wrapped myself in a silk robe. Then I put a smile on my face and turned to him.

"No, Jack. You don't owe me any more. We fell asleep. Usually that doesn't happen. It was my fault, really."

"Good, because I—" he caught himself. He got up and began putting on his clothes. I could see his mind working, considering, fitting things together and then taking them apart. "Because I'd like to see you again. For real. I mean not as a client."

I opened my mouth to tell him that it was impossible, it wouldn't work, that I didn't date my clients, that even if we started "dating," he'd always be thinking of the other men. He'd tell me that he didn't like what I did and I had to stop, and even though in my heart I knew that I already had, I couldn't bear the idea of a man wanting to have that power over me.

I opened my mouth to tell him all this, but nothing came out.

Even if I'd never seen Jack again, he still would have been my last client, but not because I'm ashamed of what I did. On the contrary. I think of the men and women I knew in my business, and I know in my heart that each one of them left my temple feeling better about themselves, about sex, about life. But I had to honor that clear voice that rang from my heart. I had to take a risk and throw myself into the universe and find another way to serve it.

Six months after that night Jack appeared at my door, I find myself in my empty Upper West Side loft—empty, that is, except for the brown moving boxes piled neatly in the center of the hardwood floor. There are fewer boxes than you would think: the expensive clothes and fancy lingerie have all been given away. I won't need them on this new journey, a journey that is taking me to another coast. To San Francisco. To a new life, and to Jack's new home.

TANTRIC EXPERIENCE

Power of Talking Dirty

Tantra supports all—light and dark. Embrace your inner bitch or bastard! Claim the power of your wholeness. Yang and yin live within. Unconditionally accept life's dualities and you transcend them.

Here is one way to add energy and power to your erotic play. Nurture the growing edge of your lovemaking by taking a walk on the wild side. Think of this as verbal S&M—you are detonating the dark dynamite of forbidden words. These words of pain and power are the blood that drips from Kali's sword.

Words like "bitch, bastard, cock, cunt, prick, pussy, fuck, shit, piss, come, tits, balls, ass, butt" are, in this society, mantras of power. You did not place the power into them, but you inherited the right to make skillful use of that power.

Are you uncomfortable with these words? A couple has to take risks together to reach new horizons of loving pleasure. If you stay with what you know, you will not have a chance to grow.

Red-hot tantra says, "Embrace the reality of release wherever it arises. While doing no harm, make use of every possible tool to arouse passionate awareness. Nothing is forbidden. Everything is permitted. The non-dual affirmation 'I am That' means I am anything and everything. I am All."

How did I discover the world of dirty sex talk? She made me do it. Honest.

I started out my short-lived but glorious relationship with Roxanne saying something like "Hey, baby, you're so beautiful. You're a goddess! Let's make love." I'd smile and try to show that I was sweet and harmless—a real nice guy.

She spit my nice guy strategy right back in my face. "What do you mean, little boy? You want to fuck me, you selfish bastard? Huh? You want to stick that big hard dick into my hot little pink wet pussy? Huh?" She licked her finger and put it in inside her, then licked it again. "Hmm. That's good! Oh shit, that is so fucking good."

I quickly discovered that this kind of talk made me want to fuck my hot nasty little bitch now, and hard! Yet when I made my move towards her in response to her erotic display, she'd back away from me and say "You're pathetic! You don't fucking deserve me!"

But if I appeared to lose interest, she turned it up another notch. She was an accomplished mistress of dirty sex talk. I was but her humble student. By the way, after all that build-up, she did deliver the goods. She was not just a tease.

Here are some practical pointers from my foul-mouthed mentor:

(1) Repeat, repeat, repeat. Example: "Oh, god, that's good. Oh, shit, that's good. Oh, my god, my pussy feels sooo ... fuckinggg ... good!" Groupings of three are especially effective.

(2) Establish a rhythm, a repetitious cadence with your words. For example, you could say "Yeah, lover, come here and fuck me. Yeah, fuck me! Fuck me, hot stuff. Fuck, fuck, fuck me. Fuck me now! Now! I need you so bad!" Only one dirty word was used over and over.

(3) Reinforce your words with dramatic bodily action. Roxanne did the sizzling tongue-to-finger thing.

I don't care how many times you see it done—it still works!

(4) Vary your volume and tonality. Roxanne went from a low, husky growl—"You think you deserve me?"—to a high-pitched ecstatic scream-moan— "Oh God, that feels so fucking good!"

(5) Create a tempo of subtle psychological torture, of yes-no, yes-no, *yes-no!* This is very effective with men. It drives them crazy with desire. It is probably less useful with women.

(6) Don't be afraid to evoke a little anger. Anger, aggression, and hot sex are hard-wired into each other, more so for some lovers than others. Yes, this is a controversial issue! Yes, if the game leads to actual violence, it went too far! I speak here only of "verbal violence," aural aggression—not physical harm!

There is a huge sexual charge hidden away in those nasty little four-letter words. That nuclear energy is yours for the taking.

The ancient wisdom of tantra clearly asserts this challenging truth: To claim your pleasure, you must claim your power. There is no other path.

I know from living my life in the tantric spirit one thing is true: Tantra is not about being nice. It is about being real. Totally real.

Take a moment to review the hottest, sexiest scenes in novels, on television, and in movies. You will find that dirty talk gave many great sex scenes the raw edge that took them over the top and made them memorable, not just for the characters, but for you as well.

In the story, Alison and Jack discover that "dirty" can refer to the rich, fresh, unspoiled soil out of which new love and life grow as well as culturally imposed notions of right and wrong. For love to be real, it must be fresh.

Sometimes, the path to renewing that freshness takes you over strange bridges into the unknown. These transitions make sense to you only after you have crossed them and looked back.

The paradox of love is that the heart expands by breaking. Only when it has been broken so often and so totally that it cannot close does it then stay wide open to everyone and everything. Then it knows the tantra, then it is living love, and not before. No pain, no gain.

There is no life without death, no pain without pleasure, no beautiful words without ugly words. The one needs the other like the day needs the night. To run from harshness in the pursuit of prettiness is to live condemned to the surface of things, for the truth can be found only in the roots, hidden deep in dark, rich, dangerous soil. The plant that flourishes grows the fruits of paradox.

CHAPTER SEVEN

7

TANTRIC BREATHING

TANTRIC TALE

Energy Orgasm

DANIEL CREEPS INTO THE ROOM AT TEN MINUTES TO EIGHT and sees that it's almost filled by thirty or so people sitting on low, round floor cushions. Daniel finds an empty cushion in the back, sits down awkwardly and glances around. He'd expected a lot of gray ponytails and peasant dresses, but instead, despite a prevalence of sweat pants and t-shirts, the crowd looks like they should be out partying on a Friday night, not sitting in wood-floored yoga studio. There are all ages, races and combinations: white, black, Asian, Indian, gay, straight. Out of habit, he scans the women for possibilities. He catches the eye of an almond-eyed girl with silky black hair and sculpted cheekbones, but she only gives him a friendly smile before turning her gaze to the empty chair at the front of the room. He feels guilty, like he's been caught thinking dirty thoughts in church.

Why had he come? He thinks of the flyer at home on his coffee table. Under a photo of a stocky man in his fifties were the words:

> "Like a key unlocking a secret door to hidden treasure, outer stimuli release pleasurable feelings

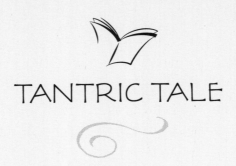

> from an inner storehouse. Alcohol, coitus, cocaine, getting a raise, winning an award—the outer stimuli are many; the source of pleasure is one. The source of pleasure is within you."

In truth, Daniel had thought it was an ad for a masturbation workshop, and his curiosity had gotten the better of him. As if he really needs a workshop on how to masturbate. He beats off in the shower on a regular basis—just to relieve stress, if nothing else. Not that finding a partner would be a problem: his voicemail is full of messages from beautiful, willing women. A voice in his head pipes up: *And you're sick of all of them.* He tells the voice to shut the fuck up.

The room stirs, and Daniel looks up to see the man from the flyer. He wears a red silk robe that reaches his knees; as he turns to adjust his chair, Daniel sees that the back of the robe is embroidered with a Hindu god and goddess intertwined in a sex act. The teacher sits, gazes out at the assembled crowd and smiles. Then he closes his eyes, resting his hands on his thighs.

Suddenly, the full impact of where he is hits Daniel. Is he about to see some old guy masturbate in front of thirty people? Daniel looks for the door. There's still time to bolt.

And then there's not. A young, wiry man in cargo pants speaks from the back of the room. "Hi, everyone. We're about to shut the doors, and we won't be opening them for the next twenty minutes. During that time, if you do need to leave, please do so, but we ask that you not re-enter and instead come back next week. Thanks." He pulls the doors closed.

There's no way that Daniel's going to call attention to himself by leaving now. As the young man passes, Daniel taps him.

"Dude, I ..." He's not sure what to say.

The young man gives Daniel a friendly smile. "Is this your first time here?"

"Yeah."

"I'll explain," says a female voice next to Daniel. He turns to see, on the cushion next to him, a beautiful black woman. He doesn't even remember seeing her sit down.

"Thanks, Josephine."

Josephine pulls her cushion close to Daniel, so close that they are almost touching. She wears saffron-colored yoga pants and a matching top, her sculpted features set off by a crown of curls pulled into a ponytail atop her head. Daniel can't tell her age. There isn't a line on her face. She radiates serenity.

"I don't know why I'm here," Daniel blurts out.

She smiles. "If you're here, you're supposed to be here."

Although the rest of the room is quiet, Josephine's voice is so low and soft that only Daniel can hear it. It lulls him, and he feels calmer, though his skin is buzzing. In fact, it seems to him that the entire room is buzzing, even though no one else is speaking or moving. The teacher's chest rises and falls under his robe.

"It isn't obvious, but he's using a special breathing technique," Josephine says. "He's taking a long, deep inhale, then breathing out even deeper and longer. The ratio between his inbreath and his outbreath is about one to two.

"But his secret is actually an energy center located in his lower abdomen. This sensitive point is below his navel, about two inches above the pubic hairline. This is the gateway to sexual pleasure. Everyone has one, but unlike most of us, he doesn't need a partner to feel it. He doesn't even need to touch his genitals or become erect to enter into a state of orgasm."

"How is that possible?" Daniel whispers.

"He's learned how to intensify the pleasurable feeling by pressing down with the muscles in the lower belly as he breathes out. This encourages the flow of pleasure. He does this every time he exhales, keeping his tongue touching the roof of his mouth."

Daniel wants to ask questions, but he keeps his mouth shut and his eyes on the teacher. Even from the back of the room, he can hear the gentle, rasping sounds of the man's breath. A chime sounds in a corner of the room. Daniel glances at his watch. It's five minutes to eight.

Josephine continues. "Now he changes his focus from spreading the energy to stacking it. He's imagining three white inner tubes—the kind you float on a lazy river—stacked on top of each other. They completely encircle his body.

"Do you see how he's intensifying his breathing? He's filling up the first inner tube. It corresponds to the first chakra, the root energy center located at the base of the spine. He's visualizing this root energy as an inflatable, sensitive ring circling his body at the level of the tail bone."

Daniel watches as the teacher pauses, then continues breathing. His stomach presses out against his robe.

"Now he's filling the second tube," says Josephine. "He imagines that it surrounds and is inflated by the sexual pleasure center, which includes his genitals and extends an inch above his pubic hairline. When he's filled this second tube, he goes back to the first one and makes sure it's still full."

Daniel only half hears Josephine's voice. *That's enough,* he thinks. He just wants to watch the teacher.

"Now he has two fully inflated imaginary inner tubes around his body filled with his breath energy. He maintains the rhythmic tightening of the lower belly muscles with each exhalation. Each time he breathes out, he encourages deeper pleasure."

Daniel can't keep quiet any longer. "Isn't this hard to do?" he whispers.

"He'd tell you that nothing that feels so good is hard to do."

Daniel stares at the teacher, amazed and jealous. To have that amount of self-control! It doesn't seem possible.

"He's filling the third and last inner tube, the one around the solar plexus," Josephine continues. "Now he now has three invisible inner tubes stacked up. He tests each one to make sure it is fully inflated. Then he tests all three together.

"He's ready. He knows that when he takes the energy up to the fourth center, to the heart, his energy will explode. He takes one last deep breath, the deepest breath of all, and takes the energy up higher, to the heart."

Josephine falls silent. The chime sounds again, eight times. A soft, lucid silence follows, as if snow is falling in the room.

Suddenly, the teacher's body stiffens and then explodes in what seems to be an ecstatic frenzy of groans and cries. He throws his head back and forth, and pounds the floor with his feet, his arms flailing. Daniel sees the whites of his eyes as they roll back in their sockets.

"Oh, God!" the teacher screams. "Oh, my God!"

Daniel sits rooted to his cushion, pinned there by the shock waves of energy coming from the man. It has to be real. These are the sounds that only lovers make, that he himself has made on a very few occasions. But never in his thirty-two years has he experienced what this man seems to be experiencing. Daniel's heart pounds; his own penis stirs.

"How long does this go on?" Daniel whispers. His mouth is dry.

"About twenty minutes."

Daniel looks at his watch: ten after eight.

Tears flow from the teacher's eyes as he continues to moan. Bliss seems to vibrate through his body like the aftershocks of an earthquake. His robe has fallen open, showing his heaving chest and round belly. *He looks like a statue of the smiling Buddha,* Daniel thinks, and then with embarrassment remembers that the last time he saw such a statue was in a bar that served twelve-dollar martinis.

"Those are tears of joy," Josephine says. Her face glows. "Tears of yearning. Of heartache."

All of which Daniel has experienced, but not for a very long time. The face of his college girlfriend—the first and last time he ever cried over a woman—flashes through his mind. A spasm contracts his heart. *I'm not going to cry*, he tells himself. But his eyes are wet. He glances at his watch again: 8:15. Five minutes left.

"I guess this is how he gets his exercise," Daniel whispers, regretting the words the instant they leave his mouth. But Josephine just gives him a sympathetic look.

The silence in the room begins to disturb Daniel. How can everyone sit so still with this display? He wants to leave. Why can't he? He wants to go home and jerk off until he can forget what he's seeing, even though he knows, suddenly, that he wouldn't be able to stand the pathetic orgasm that would result—not when he's seen what's possible. It would be like eating packaged doughnuts for dinner when a magnificent meal of meat and bread, fruit and wine, covers the next table. Josephine reaches over and takes his hand, like a mother calming a child.

The teacher's movements slow, calm. His moans die down; his breathing steadies. A flush has seeped across his chest and neck.

His face radiates serenity and joy, as though he'd acquired a spiritual tan.

Even though Daniel's never seen someone enter the afterglow state—if he paid attention to his lovers, he might have, but he's usually flat on his back enjoying his own post-climax bliss—he know that this is what he's seeing now. The teacher's climax was real. Envy washes over Daniel once again. To feel that sense of peace, if only for a few minutes!

He glances around. The others in the room haven't taken their attention from the teacher. They seem to have been meditating, riding the waves of the teacher's energy to their own inner paradises. Could he ever learn to do this?

The teacher opens his eyes, and casts his arms wide in a gesture of blessing. He smiles, his eyes glowing. Then he pantomimes lighting a post-coital cigarette.

"Damn, I'm good!" he says.

Laughter ripples through the room. People begin to move and stretch. Josephine leans over to Daniel. "He always makes this joke."

"What happens now?"

"People ask questions. He'll give some beginning instructions for the energy orgasm master technique and talk about upcoming workshops." She touches Daniel's arm. "You've had a lot to absorb. It's all right if you leave."

Daniel wants to stay, but he feels drained. "OK. Thanks."

He slips out of the room as quietly as he slipped in, and the cold night air hits him like a slap in the face. He realizes that he has not done something that would normally be a reflex: he has not asked Josephine for her number, nor does he have any desire to. But he does want to be in her presence again. In the teacher's presence. He wants to be in that room again. The thought hits him like an electric shock.

"That was stupid," he says out loud. "I'm not going back."

But already, he knows that he will, just as he knows that he won't be joining his friends at the martini bar tonight. He'd thought he'd have a good story for them. Now, he just wants to go home and think about the teacher in the red robe. He wants to count the days until next Friday night.

TANTRIC EXPERIENCE

Easy Energy Orgasm

THE TECHNIQUE USED BY THE TEACHER IN THE STORY IS identical to the one I used to demonstrate the energy orgasm to workshop participants in the United States and Canada as well as on the Playboy Channel.

I have used this method to successfully demonstrate an energy climax lasting for up to twenty minutes for groups of five to seventy. Stacking the inner tubes of energy is my unique technique.

The instructions work. With practice, you, too, will be able to have an internal energy orgasm experience whenever you like.

Practice first on your back. Keep your knees up, your feet flat on the ground. That is how I started. I took a class at a new age health fair. The small room was jammed with forty people. Other people's feet were in my face!

I learned the rudiments of energy climaxing by doing Reichian and Native American breathwork. In those systems, you rock back and forth from the pelvis as you breathe deeply into your lower belly while lying on your back. You will find more information on these approaches in the Red Hot Resources section of this book.

The secret key is to learn how to feel pleasure in the sex center at the lower belly only from the breathing and the muscle contractions. This is not easy. It takes practice. Disciplines such as yoga and chi kung may help.

I sit on a chair for demonstrations, but not at home (if for no other reason than the very real risk of falling and hurting myself). I start out sitting cross-legged on a pillow, tuning into and feeling the pleasure center in my lower belly. I get my energy going by swaying side to side and rocking back and forth. Although I don't need music, it makes it more fun. I prefer rock or funk—music with a strong beat.

You cannot force this energy orgasm technique. You must first locate and sensitize the lower belly center. Once you achieve this, you have activated the energy orgasm potential of your body. You will be able to feel pleasure radiating out from this center and streaming through the body with each breath.

You are simply *allowing* this to happen. Again, you cannot force it as an act of will. Nor do you need to imagine it. Fine-tune your ability to directly feel—that means no intervening thoughts, images or concepts—the sensations in the lower belly. With practice, you will discover that the pleasure is already there. It is native to the body. It may help to think of this sensing skill as *touching* that area with your mind or attention.

If you have difficulty locating this special spot, therapist Jack Johnston offers an excellent step-by-step approach in his guide *Male Multiple Orgasm* (see Red Hot Resources). This title is somewhat misleading, as his systematic approach will help women as well as men achieve the delights of internal orgasm ecstasy.

As described in the story, the ratio of the in-breath to the out-breath is two to one. This means that your exhalation takes *at least* twice as long. It may take three or four times as long as it grows more refined during your inner ecstasy meditation session.

However, this result should occur naturally as the meditation progresses and you go deeper into the energy orgasm state. At no time should there be a feeling of strain or struggle in what you are doing. With all energy techniques that involve breathing, there is an element of risk if the technique is forced.

When you exhale, really pull in the lower abdomen. As you do this, feel this area from deep within the body. It is as if you are stroking it with your attention from the inside to make it come alive. If you are doing this contraction properly, you will feel your anal muscles tighten as well.

Once you are able to generate pleasurable feeling in the lower belly center, graduate to building the inner energy air tubes. This technique is as simple as it sounds. However, it is not just a mental picture. You must *feel* that you are literally filling the tubes up with air, with energy, exactly as if they are physical inner tubes, the kind that children swim around in at a lake or in a pool.

Visualize and feel the first tube, fat and round, circling all the way around your body at the level of your tailbone. Fill this tube up until it feels completely full, even stuffed to the point of nearly exploding. You need to be experiencing this full feeling first before moving on to the second tube.

The second tube is stacked on top of the first tube. This means you need to remember to keep the first tube filled to its limit while you are filling up the second tube. The second tube goes over the sex center and the lower belly pleasure point.

The third tube rests on top of the second. Now you must keep both lower tubes full as you fill up this one surrounding the navel. Remember, it goes all the way around your body, so you will seem to feel it at your lower back, too.

This sounds more complicated than it really is. Yes, once you master it, it will be as easy as riding a bike. Unless you are tired and very low energy, stacking these three energy tubes around the body is fun, easy and uplifting.

The first tube fills up the root chakra to capacity and overflowing. The second tube has the same effect on the second or sex chakra. The third tube maximizes the third chakra energy level. In this way, all three lower chakras are filled to bursting with energy. They are overflowing, which creates an ideal launching pad for the internal energy. The only direction it can now go is up.

You feel charged-up, yet suspended in time and space. You are in a "pregnant pause," the calm before the chaos of bliss breaks you wide open and sends you soaring out of control into the joy of the vastness. Your anticipation is accelerating. You are filled with a magnificent invisible potential, and it is now going to reveal itself. Yet you are not sure what to expect!

Here comes the moment you have been waiting for. Closing your eyes, invite into your heart your yearnings for love, for ecstasy, for bliss, for fusion with the divine, for complete surrender, for total let-go. These are deep yearnings of the human heart, of every heart, and they can be called upon at will.

As these feelings gather in the fourth chakra, they create a vacuum through vulnerability. An urgent spiritual call goes out from the core of your being. Yet this sense of emptiness, of divine discontentment, is a positive acknowledgment of your deeper yearning for wholeness. This sincere aspiration draws the energy up from the lower chakras into the heart center.

By earnestly feeling, and not just thinking about, the yearnings of your heart, an internal explosion occurs. The energy spontaneously leaps up to the heart chakra. The heart chakra is a realm of higher vibration, one in which pure bliss can be felt from within without any stimulation other than your own internal willingness and free attention.

From there, it naturally goes up your spine to your third eye, to your crown and through the top of your head to the light, love and wide-open bright space above it. If you do not find yourself spontaneously doing the Tibetan Eye Roll when the energy jumps up to the heart, then do the Roll and lean your head back slightly, as if swooning. The energy should then effortlessly go all the way up.

This may sound abstract, but when you actually do it, it won't be. An invisible lover is making love to you, carrying you higher and higher. You reach the cosmic heart of space. It is right there, above your head. You cannot believe all of this glory lives inside of you. Your mind is struck speechless. Your heart swells with rapture and melts with gratitude.

Please persist with this energy orgasm technique. You will achieve amazing union with this blissful, loving reality!

After resting at this pinnacle, you may experience a shower of blessings as the erotic spiritual ecstasy rains down all around and through your body from the cosmic center up above. Encourage this sweet, healing rain to permeate your body in every cell.

Once you have learned how to do it, you can access this ecstatic experience any time you like. When I first discovered how to do the energy orgasm, I did it five times a day every day for two months!

For some reason, my public energy orgasm demonstrations are quite dramatic. Perhaps it is my secret desire to be the center of attention—at last, they're going to have to look at me now!

By the way, people can feel the energy at my live shows. After I gave a demonstration to more than seventy seminar attendees in Toronto, I asked the group, "Do you believe that was real? Or do you think I faked it?"

A man and a woman in the front row I did not know volunteered "Oh, no, we know it was real. We could feel the bliss along with you."

Finally, to say it is "on tap like beer" is not completely accurate. When I was doing it five times a day, I found that the experience varied in intensity. After five repetitions, I really didn't want any more.

Also, it usually takes at least a minute or so to get the sensations going. Sometimes it takes even longer. And sometimes I just can't get my energy up to do it at all—a sort of "energy orgasm impotence"!

People have asked me, "Is it as satisfying as a regular genital climax?"

My final answer is "Yes!"

The sensations are not as sharply physical and localized, but they are intensely pleasurable. The feelings during and after the peak climax moment are very similar to my conventional sex experiences. The rushing sensations are more ethereal. However, they are not any less pleasurable and always include my whole body, fusing it into one grinning, glowing human light bulb of erotic joy.

There is an emotional component to sexual pleasure and orgasm. It is noticed when it is lacking, whether with masturbation or intercourse. When I do my energy orgasm technique, I feel saturated with a deep emotional satisfaction as if I have just made love to a higher being. There is no feeling of lack.

You may experience "kriyas." These are spontaneous purifying movements such as head shaking or twitches. Kriyas are quite common. These spontaneous movements are caused by kundalini. Surrender to them. You will discover these releases feel good. You may even begin to look forward to them. You will find detailed information about kriyas at the comprehensive kundalini Web sites listed in Red-Hot Resources.

I am convinced that doing this energy orgasm technique is a gentle, thrilling way to safely awaken kundalini and effortlessly dance to higher spiritual levels. I have tremendous confidence in the safety as well as the effectiveness of this energy orgasm technique. Please let me know of your wonderful experiences at my Web site www.redhottantra.com. Enjoy!

Finally, I invite you to ask yourself some deeper questions. These questions are at the heart of spiritual tantra. Self-discovery is the highest ecstasy.

- Am I scared of bliss? Do I find pleasure threatening?
- Does the true source of my bliss live within me?
- If I celebrate and integrate both yang and yin within, what happens to my need to be completed by others? Will I live from unconditional love more?

In the story, a group of gifted individuals embrace energy orgasm as part of their spiritual path. They find that through direct experience their questions are answered at a level beyond the mind. Such is the way of tantra.

Perhaps you will be like Daniel. Having experienced a vicarious taste of the innate ecstasy, you will want to come back for more.

Try it. You just might like it!

TANTRIC TALE

Breath of Fire

I'M STANDING IN MY OFFICE—THAT IS, THE CORNER OF OUR bedroom where I have my desk—when I realize how much I hate my calendar. Sure, it seems benign enough, what with its photographs of waterfalls, sunsets and all that nature crap I suppose is meant to be soothing. But the pretty pictures don't distract me from the thirty or so squares marching across the lower half of the page, squares filled with handwriting that tell me my husband and I have no time to ourselves. Doctor's appointments. Conference calls. Play dates for our three-year-old Jack. All those filled-up squares send a clear message: This calendar belongs to someone who has no time to fuck. And that's why I hate it. Why can't there be just one empty square? Just one square that I can fill with a single word: SEX.

Mike chooses this moment to wander in, announcing his entrance by stumbling over one of Jack's wooden toy trucks. I glance at the clock on my nightstand. It's ten P.M., which means Mike will just be getting started on answering e-mail from his "office," a corner in the living room of our tiny, two-bedroom apartment. And me? Other than hating my calendar, I'm ready for bed.

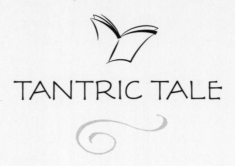

"No one told me that being a parent meant you're constantly stubbing your toe on tiny hard objects," Mike says, pushing the truck to one side.

"Do you know we haven't had sex in three weeks?" I tell him.

"What? Let me see that." He takes the calendar from me.

"The last time we had sex was the weekend we were at the beach."

Now we're both staring at the calendar as if it were an oracle. Which it is. "Three weeks," he says. "Christ." He rubs the stubble on his jaw, as if the answer could be found in facial hair.

"Do you want to have sex?" I ask.

"Right now?"

"Yes."

He glances at his watch. "How about in an hour?"

I can't decide whether I'm pissed or relieved. "I'll be asleep in an hour."

We look at each other. I love Mike, and I know he loves me, but right now I feel like if we didn't ever have sex again, it wouldn't be the end of the world.

"What's happened to us?" I say. "We used to have sex all the time. I mean, *all* the time. Now I don't even think about it."

One week later, I've just gotten Jack to fall asleep when Mike calls to me from his computer. I come into the kitchen ready to kill him for making so much noise, but the excited look on his face stops me.

"Honey, listen to this," he says. "There's a name for what we have. ISD. Inhibited sexual desire."

I go to the kitchen sink and turn on the water. Part of me finds his enthusiasm utterly adorable, but the other part is too pissed off at him. He's let the dishes pile up in the sink yet again, and after two days, I can't stand it any more.

"There's a name for it?" I ask. "I just thought we didn't want to fuck."

I know this isn't quite fair. Deep down, I'm touched that he's actually looked up our "problem."

"But I *do* want to fuck," he says. He looks back at the computer. "It says that ISD is a 'very common sexual disorder.' It says the most common cause 'seems to be relationship problems where one partner does not feel emotionally intimate or close to their mate.' Is that it? You don't feel close to me?" He comes over and tries to nuzzle me.

I hold up a dripping plate that holds the remnants of last night's pizza dinner.

"You don't want to fuck me because I left dishes in the sink?" he asks.

"News flash: resentment is not an aphrodisiac."

"Okay, Okay. I'll be better about doing my dishes. Give me those sexy rubber gloves right now."

"It's not just that, honey. It seems like we never talk. I can't remember the last time we had a real conversation. Remember that night when we were first dating, and you brought over a bottle of wine, and we sat on the patio and talked for hours? Now I'm always tired, and you're always working."

"What are we going to do about it?" There's worry in his dark brown eyes.

"Deb and Phil had this problem. I should ask them."

"Deb and Phil? *Sex maniacs* Deb and Phil? Christ, if you can believe them, they're *always* having sex. I don't see how they have time to work and raise kids."

"If I found out what they did, would you try it with me?"

"Sure, why not?"

He's just leaned in to kiss me when we hear a cry from Jack's bedroom. "Mommy, I'm thirsty!" our son wails.

I look at Mike. "I'm making that call tomorrow."

And that's how we find ourselves sitting in the waiting room of a tantric sex therapist. It looks like a regular doctor's office. There's even a ficus in the corner. The only hint that there's something different about this doctor is the reading material. Instead of *People* and *National Geographic,* we've got magazines like *Shambala Sun* and *Yoga Journal.* Mike nervously flips through a copy of *Tricycle.*

"Tell me why we're here again?" he asks without looking up. "This guy really helped Deb and Phil?"

I realize that he's terrified.

"It's okay, honey," I tell him, taking his hand. "We're not going to have to have sex in front of him."

He gives me the deer-in-the-headlights look and is just about to answer, no doubt to tell me he's leaving, when the door opens and a middle-aged man comes into the waiting room.

"Mike? Alisa? I'm Benjamin Sullivan."

Benjamin is a round man of medium height, with friendly blue eyes, and dark hair and beard. With his plaid shirt and pleated khaki pants, he is exactly what you would picture if someone said the word "therapist." He is exactly *not* what you would picture if someone said, "*tantric sex* therapist."

Benjamin leads us into his office, and we sink into a plush leather couch lined with silk cushions as he sits in a large armchair opposite us. I glance around the room. The shelves are lined with the standard psychology texts I've seen in my own therapist's office, but I also notice books on Hinduism, tantra, and Zen Buddhism. On his desk is an orchid in a celadon blue pot, and a small statue of a naked woman sitting on a man's lap, her legs wrapped around him. I try not to stare at it.

"What can I do for you two?" Benjamin asks.

"We have ISD," Mike blurts out.

Benjamin smiles. "What makes you think that?"

"We love each other, but we just don't seem to be interested in sex anymore."

"And why do you think that is?"

We both start talking at once, and within twenty minutes, we've told Benjamin the most intimate details of our sex lives. Or lack thereof. Benjamin simply listens and nods way past the point where *I* would have gotten bored with us. Finally, we run out of steam. It seems like forever before he speaks.

"So at one point, you felt a lot of desire for each other. And when you have sex, you still enjoy it."

"Absolutely," we answer in unison.

"Well, clearly you have a lot of affection for each other. What you do not have, by the way, is ISD."

"We don't?" Mike looks almost disappointed. He hates to be wrong.

"No. ISD only applies when you've gone for six months or more without having sex, or if one or both of you was clinically depressed. What you have is a two-career marriage and a toddler. It's no wonder you're too exhausted for sex. Luckily, you've called attention to the problem early, before it develops into ISD, which can be very hard to resolve.

"Here's the good news: you've already got four out of what I call the five 'C's': compatibility, communication, consciousness, and commitment. These are all critically important for making a relationship work."

"What's the fifth?" I ask. Leave it to me to zero in on the bad news.

"Chemistry. It's not that you don't have it. It just seems like your tank is a little low, which isn't surprising or unusual. It shouldn't be hard to fill it up again. I'm going to suggest that for the next few weeks, you reserve one night a week for just the two of you. A date night. Can you find someone to watch your son for a few hours?"

"Sure," Mike says.

"Good. Go to dinner, or for a walk. I don't want you to go to a movie or do anything that involves having your focus on anything other than each other. Now, on one of these date nights, can you find someone to keep your son overnight?"

"I suppose," I say, thinking of what I'll tell my mom.

"Because the technique I'm about to explain to you will require your full attention," he says. "I think you'll find it's like pouring gasoline on a fire."

That Friday night, Mike and I sit on the bed cross-legged, facing each other. I've lit a bunch of candles, and from the corner of the room comes the sound of my favorite massage CD.

"Am I sitting right?" he asks. "What do I do with my hands?"

"Yeah. Just sit like we do at the end of yoga class."

I put my hands palms-up and touch my third finger to my thumb. He copies me—a little melodramatically, I think—and looks into my eyes. A smile twitches at the corners of his lips. He begins to snicker.

"What's so funny?"

"What if I fart?" He bursts out laughing and falls back onto the bed.

I can't help it. I start to laugh, too. "Then I'll run screaming from the room. C'mon, honey. Let's give it a try."

"Okay, okay. What do we do first?"

We face each other again, and I glance at the little note card I've put beside us. "Breathe in. Hold it. Then exhale completely and pull in your stomach."

We try this a few times, then add the next step: When we breathe out, we pull our stomachs up and in as quickly as we can. I notice that the area below Mike's ribcage hollows out. It's pretty cool. After we do this a couple of times, I realize that I'm actually feeling a little bit of a head rush, like when I stand up too fast, but it's much more pleasurable.

"Whoa," Mike says.

"I know. You ready?"

"Yeah. Through the nose."

I nod. We pull in our stomachs as we breathe out, but we do it fast, ten times, exhaling through our noses. Then we inhale and hold it. We look at each other, and go back to breathing normally. I'm definitely having the head rush feeling again, but I'm warm and tingling all over as well. My eyes settle on Mike's lap.

He's got a huge erection.

The sight of his erect penis sends an instant rush of warmth between my legs. I reach forward and slide my hand around his hardness, giving it a couple of quick strokes. He closes his eyes and gives a little moan. I think of the little statue of the intertwined man and woman on Benjamin's desk, and uncrossing my legs, I scoot up onto Mike's lap. He slips easily inside me, and his eyes fly open.

"Oh my God. You're so wet. When did that happen?"

"I don't know," I say. I don't care.

We begin to move together, our arms wrapped around each other. Mike thrusts up into me as I rock my pelvis against him. Our tongues intertwine and tease each other. It's been a long time since we made love like this. But then, after about five minutes, something Benjamin says slides its way back into my mind.

"Honey, he said we were supposed to take a break and do it again."

"What? Are you kidding?"

"No. Stop moving for a second."

He groans, but obeys. To reward him, I keep my legs wrapped tight around him and kiss his lips and neck, trailing my tongue up around his earlobes.

"You're not making this easier."

"Sorry. Ready? Go!"

We exhale quickly through our noses ten times, then inhale and hold it. My whole body begins to tingle again, from my hair to my toes and to the place where Mike fills me. Heat emanates from his skin. I feel as horny for him as I did the first time we made love, and I start moving up and down on him once more, gaining speed, as he thrusts into me. I ride him faster and faster, rubbing myself against his pubic bone. The room around me fades. I see only him.

"God, I love you," I gasp.

"I love you too," he says back. "I want you to come."

I put his hand on mine, and together we rub my clit until I feel the orgasm begin in my toes and shoot up my body. I realize that I'm screaming, and that Mike is coming, too.

Afterwards, as I lie on top of him trying to catch my breath, I hear him laughing softly.

"Now I see why Benjamin told us to have someone take Jack overnight," he says. "When can we try this again?"

"Benjamin said only once per night."

"How many hours until tomorrow night?"

We can't leave Jack with my mom every night, so we start to act like a couple of kids, trying to sneak off and have sex when our parents aren't looking. Only instead of our parents, we have a three-year-old. Over the next week, naptime, bedtime, and play dates all become opportunities to practice Benjamin's breathing technique—which he calls "Fire Breath" for good reason—and then fall on each other like cats in heat. I fall in love again, not only with my husband but with my calendar, because every appointment means either a chance to fuck undisturbed, or a challenge to be surmounted, which makes the sex even hotter. The dishes pile up in the sink. E-mails go unread. Neither of us seems to care.

We start trying out a few things that Benjamin told us were more advanced. If someone had told me a week ago that I'd be sitting on my husband's lap with his penis deep inside me and our foreheads pressed together as we hummed away, I would have asked them what they were smoking. Now I'd tell them that I'd found something better than any drug.

One night, Mike is going at me from behind, one finger on my clit as he uses his other hand to pull my hips against him. I feel like I'm flying. But then my eyes notice the bedside table—and the phone.

"Oh shit," I say.

"What's wrong?" Mike gasps behind me. "Are you okay? Did I hurt you?" He slows his movements, which is too bad, because I sensed I was starting up the delicious path to orgasm.

"We were supposed to call Benjamin. Tell him how we were doing. Set up another appointment."

"Forget it." He flips me over on my back and plunges in to me again. I lift my legs high and grab his butt, pulling him into me. How had I forgotten the feeling of him inside me? I want to keep making love to him all night, until the sun rises.

"We should call him and thank him," I whisper. My handsome husband smiles down at me, his eyes full of love and lust.

"Later," he says.

He lowers his mouth to my nipples. I take a deep breath. And hold it.

TANTRIC EXPERIENCE

Fire Breath Practice Tips

THE FIRST STEP TO SUCCESS WITH THE FIRE BREATH (BREATH of Fire) is to know how to breathe with your belly. You may already do that, but most people don't.

The yoga word for breath exercise is "pranayama." The spiritual techniques collectively called pranayama were originally designed to invoke the event of enlightenment, a state in which conventional identification with the physical body is dissolved. Unity with the conscious ocean of prana is attained. Life is then effortlessly lived from a higher, neutral, intuitive point of view.

Lie on your back with your knees up. Place a weight on your belly, such as a sand bag or a hefty book, like one of those big computer books—I'm looking at *Using HTML 4* right now on my shelf—nothing too uncomfortable or heavy, of course.

Your goal is to lift the big book or sand bag on your belly when you breathe in, then let your belly collapse, gently and under your control, when you breathe out. If you are a chest breather, as most people are, this will be a new experience for you.

If you find this exercise is difficult for you, practice it a few times first. You won't be able to do the Fire Breath properly until you have the belly movement right.

In sitting position, breathe in deeply, letting the belly expand. Hold for a moment. Now exhale completely. In order to facilitate a complete exhalation, purse your lips and breathe out of your mouth until no more air comes out. Pull your belly in as you do this.

Repeat this all-in breath, all-out breath a few times until you get the hang of it.

Now comes the interesting part. Do the same all-in breath, but when you do the all-out exhalation, now pull up and in as deeply and forcibly as you can. Don't strain yourself, of course!

Unless you have done this before, the Pull-Up should be a new experience for you. You will develop a new appreciation of your "guts."

To do the Pull-Up properly, you do not only pull in. You try to suck your belly up under your rib cage. Also, you tighten your anal muscles. If you are doing this properly, you will feel the action of your back muscles. You will also feel your lower belly muscles pulling in firmly.

Remember, first breathe in deeply, then exhale completely, and then do the Pull-Up. If you try to do the Pull-Up without completing a breath cycle, it will not have the same feeling or effect.

After you are comfortable with this technique, hold the exhalation for a few seconds. If you are doing the Pull-Up correctly, then you will probably find that it brings pleasant, uplifting feelings—even a subtle thrill. In other words, it produces a natural high!

Some sources also credit this technique with the power to help keep a person young. I know one thing for sure—getting good at the Pull-Up will help you achieve the Energy Orgasm. The point at the lower belly where you are pulling in is the secret pleasure center responsible for creating the internal orgasm experience. The subtle thrill you are feeling is a gentle, controlled, upwardly mobile kundalini rush.

While you are holding in the state of exhalation, do a mental check of these four points: (1) anus, (2) lower belly, (3) stomach sucked up inside of rib cage, (4) sitting tall with spine lengthened and lower back engaged. All should be tight and strong.

As you gain mastery with the Pull-Up, you can add the final touches: place the tip of the tongue at the roof of the mouth, and roll your eyes back into your head. Your eyes are locked in place, looking at the third eye in the center of the forehead.

You may also discover a natural tendency to tuck the chin in and down slightly. This is fine. This is the Chin-Lock. However, do not exaggerate this. You should find that this lock occurs without your effort, provided you are doing the rest of the elements of the Pull-Up properly. You will sense how it is helping to unify the exercise and pull the energy up the spine to the head.

The classic yoga name for the Pull-Up technique is "uddiyana bandha." A variation is taught in the Five Tibetans, a popular energy routine (see Red Hot Resources at the back of this book).

This is a very powerful technique. Please do not overdo it!

You may feel pleasantly light-headed for up to a few minutes after doing the Pull-Up. If this feeling persists, then you are doing too many repetitions. I would recommend no more than five to start out.

A side benefit of the Pull-Up is orgasmic awakening. If you don't achieve orgasm, the Pull-Up will help you have them. If you have them, the Pull-Up will make them even better. The Pull-Up strengthens and energizes the sexual nerves in the lower belly and pelvic bowl, enhancing your pleasure response.

Even if your orgasms are not cosmic, they can still make the earth move. The Pull-Up will make that a consistent fulfillment for you. Obviously, there are plenty of factors that come into play when you climax, but the Pull-Up will maximize your orgasm potential—and your orgasm potential is sky-high.

I am recommending that you practice the Pull-Up along with the Fire Breath. The Pull-Up improves your Fire Breath technique, adding power, sensitivity and feeling. Do five or ten repetitions of the Pull-Up. Then do five or ten Fire Breaths. When you're making love with Fire Breath, though, just do the Fire Breath.

Like the Pull-Up, the Fire Breath is not something you play with. Do it vigorously for just ten repetitions according to the instructions below. You will soon experience the power of the Fire Breath for yourself. You will quickly understand how it got its name!

What if you don't experience anything? Then you are probably moving the belly in and out too shallowly. That is why I taught you the Pull-Up first. You must pull in your stomach quickly, deeply and vigorously!

Done incorrectly, the Fire Breath may not seem like much—just shallow panting. Done properly, the Fire Breath is like adding gasoline to a fire! You feel vividly alive. Your whole body gets hot. You're "all fired up."

Begin by sitting up. Sitting cross-legged is fine. Breathe through the nose.

Remember the Pull-Up? Now do it very quickly, very forcibly, with a jerk. Suck in the lower belly. The gut is, more or less, going under the rib cage.

Obviously, because you are doing the Fire Breaths so quickly, you cannot get the same complete coverage of all those feeling points that you could during the Pull-Up. Now, just pull in as forcibly and as quickly as you can.

Start out slowly, making sure you are pulling all the way in with a forcible, emphatic jerk of the stomach muscles. Breathe through your nose. Begin to accelerate the speed of these movements. Do just five or ten the first time.

You will be making a sniffing sound out the nose. A common metaphor is the old steam engine—a choo-choo train. This train is going faster and faster and faster. That is what your Fire Breath will be like with a little practice. Remember, you are breathing through the nose only.

The climax of the Fire Breath is that after, say, ten repetitions, you then hold the exhalation. In yoga, you can hold the inhalation or the exhalation. After doing the Fire Breath vigorously ten times, it should feel natural to hold the exhalation or out-breath for an unusually long time. Or you can take in a deep breath and hold that.

I do both. First, I hold the out-breath. Then I take in a deep in-breath, and hold that as long as it is comfortable.

Assume the energy circulation posture practiced in the Pull-Up. Your tongue is touching the roof of your mouth. Your eyes are rolled back.

Your chin may be tucked in, or it may have floated up. I find that it may do either with me. Don't force the chin to tuck in if it doesn't want to. Never force anything while doing breathing techniques.

If you like, visualize light or listen to OM in your mind. Or just float away in the silence. This may feel quite blissful. You may experience the upward rushes of pleasant sensation mentioned earlier. You may feel more energy, more prana or life-force, in and around your body. The Fire Breath is clearing the energy channels of your body. Sooner or later, you will feel the effects.

Please do a round of Fire Breaths—five or ten "snoofs" (sniffing sounds made out the nose)—before you read the next section.

If you did your Fire Breaths with proper vigor, then you discovered that your "snoofs" will clear your nasal passages. Therefore, if you will be doing Fire Breath with a partner, blow your nose before becoming intimate!

I recommend this from personal experience. I neglected to blow my nose beforehand. I didn't feel anything in my nose, so I thought I was fine.

I did ten vigorous Fire Breaths and a big "booger" shot out my nose. Fortunately, it did not strike my partner! But she did see the nasal missile and identified its landing site on the otherwise clean white sheets. Gracefully, she was an enthusiastic yoga student and gave the Fire Breath and me a second chance!

Another fine point is that you have the option of filling up on the in-breath, or just letting the muscular jerk of the stomach at the exhalation handle the whole thing. Technically, if you don't get involved in the inhalation, and just let it happen automatically, this called "bhastrika" in classical hatha yoga. If you do Fire Breath this way, you are not incorrect. The more powerful Tantric/Sikh version is the one I prefer to do.

When you actively inhale at the in-breath, which means you will have more air force to exhale because you inhaled more air, you are doing the modern Fire Breath. The Fire Breath I have taught here has similarities to the technique taught by Yogi Bhajan's 3HO

Kundalini Yoga students. If you need more personal guidance, they offer classes and instructional videos (see Red Hot Resources).

It may help you to place one or both hands on the belly to help you focus there. This way you will have a concrete physical sensation—the contact of your hands against your belly—to give you a now-moment target. If you are having trouble keeping your focus as you do the Fire Breath, this may help.

Congratulations! Now you know how to do the Fire Breath. Now let's learn how to use it to turn up the heat during lovemaking. The Fire Breath can be performed at any time and in any position. I am thinking of times when I was on top, paused and did the Fire Breath in order to delay my ejaculation. I am also remembering moments when my partner did the Fire Breath to bring on and intensify her climax.

However, the overall approach that I recommend is to stop making love and take a Fire Breath break. This break time can be combined with eating and drinking to refuel.

If you are still in foreplay mode, then you don't need to disunite. But if you were in intercourse, you will need to separate. Then you will sit facing each other on the bed, if that's practical, and do the Fire Breath together.

It may help to sit on small, firm pillows. Another possibility, the one I ended up using, is to lounge on large, overstuffed, Moroccan-style pillows on the bed or within easy reach. Just prop these plush back-supports against the wall and lean back. Enjoy your Fire Breath break in first-class comfort.

What happens during the break? You build up and intensify your sexual energy charge, both within your body and with your partner. You also balance and harmonize your sexual energy charge. Charging up with energy is the yang side of the Fire Breath. Balancing energy is its yin function. Somehow, it manages to do both at the same time.

The outcome is delightful. The woman has more energy for her orgasms and is able to achieve states of greater whole-body pleasure. The man finds that his energy is balanced and calm, yet firm and strong. He experiences significant gains in his endurance, his so-called "staying power." In other words, the Fire Breath can make him a real stud!

Ah, but I can hear what you're thinking ... David, once I'm united with my lover, I don't want to separate again, not until we have to. Please do try the Fire Breath in combination with a refueling stop. It's fantastic for those "marathon" lovemaking sessions. However, there is a way to hold onto your oneness. It is called the Yab-Yum position.

Perhaps you have seen the Tibetan Buddhist statues of deities making love facing each other. The woman is in the man's lap. This is the Yab-Yum position.

This is the most advanced form. It assumes that you both can do the Fire Breath. By doing the Fire Breath in this position, you can stay genitally united and gain all the benefits.

I find that three Yab-Yum Fire Breath breaks is usually about right for me and my partner. It is good to designate one person as Fire Breath leader. They will start the breath by announcing "Okay, 3-2-1 ... go!" Or "Om! Om! Om!" And then you start.

This may seem too regimented, but I find that doing the breath together, including that choo-choo train acceleration, and then holding the exhalation in a meditation space, is simply fantastic. It brings you closer together in ways that are completely beyond words.

Remember, this is an ultra-powerful technique. Done together in unison, it becomes even more potent. After you complete your ten repetitions together, that's enough. That's one session. If you feel fantastic, then do another ten reps on your next break. That's it! That's plenty for your first Fire Breath workout.

Now that you've mastered Fire Breath in Yab-Yum with your partner, let's add a final, supercharging touch to it—the Cosmic Fire Breath!

In *Sexual Energy Ecstasy,* I said "Sex is nature's LSD." Twenty years later, I am still saying that. Doing the Fire Breath together, especially if you add this cosmic touch, should prove my claim beyond any doubt.

After you complete a Fire Breath session in Yab-Yum, initiate each other with a wet kiss on the forehead, at the third eye.

Or moisten your little finger and apply your saliva there. Saliva has electrochemical properties that support the subtle energetic exchange between you.

Bend forward slightly so that your foreheads are touching. Now "Hummm" out loud together. Feel the vibration through your unified third eyes. Merge in telepathic communion—one heart, one mind, one body, one spirit.

Now allow yourselves to float away, up through the crown chakra at the top of your head. Imagine a sphere of golden light there, where you unite.

If it is not too complicated, inside this golden globe see a god and goddess who, like you, are sitting in Yab-Yum. Alternatively, you can see a radiant, blissful Buddha or other enlightened figure sitting on top of your head.

Take your joined energy up and merge with your high tantric visualization. From the heart, silently invoke the love, bliss and blessings of this sacred symbol of divine perfection and wholeness.

Linger at this peak. The cosmic symbol blesses both of you and sends a stream of sweet, divine nectar down through, between and all around you.

Sink back down into your own body. Allow these luminous bliss energies to seep into, totally saturate and completely surround your physical body. Feel that you are soaked through and through by the blessed nectar.

Do not try to do this for your partner. He or she must take responsibility for absorbing the blessings into their own physical vehicle at this time.

This nectar is healing as well as grounding. Enjoy this part. Take your time. Allow this sweet sexual medicine energy to work its way all down through your body, into every cell. Let it go all the way down to and through the soles of your feet.

If purification has taken place, then toxins are being eliminated through the soles of your feet. Will these dark emissions to go hundreds or thousands of feet deep into the earth. There are entities down there for whom your energetic excrement is a delicious dessert! I mention this since psychic detoxification is likely to happen, especially the first few times you do this powerful process.

After doing any form of the Fire Breath, come down slowly. Take plenty of time to come down. Return gently and cautiously. This means you have scheduled in plenty of time for "debriefing." You do not want to have to rush to some meeting or appointment now! You have gone out of this world. Now is the reentry.

Drink plenty of water. Have a good, solid meal. Share massages. Maybe even have a cold shower. Sometimes, it is hard to recognize just how spaced out you are, as you get used to this high, expanded state. This is true for any intensive breathing work.

Especially, don't just jump into your car and drive off into the sunset—or sunrise—after an intense, high-powered, super-energy lovemaking session like this. Please exercise caution! You want to be completely back in your body before you get into your car!

Here's my true story. I walked out to the car after a beautiful session in Los Angeles that involved the Cosmic Fire Breath. I remember thinking "I feel fantastic!" And I did. But feeling good isn't everything.

I had parked the car on an incline. It was a stick shift. I put the car into neutral. Then, in a daze, I watched as several telephone poles rolled past me. "That sure is strange," I said out loud. "Why are those telephone poles moving?"

Remember, I had not been drinking or taking drugs! I was so out of it, so naturally "high," that I could not recognize that I had put the car in neutral and it was now rolling backwards! Fortunately, my car went only a short distance and bumped into a trashcan. However, you may not be as lucky as I was.

That's the Cosmic Fire Breath in Yab-Yum. It is a top tantric secret. I have included details here that you will not find anywhere else. I guarantee that it will, to use the vernacular of the sixties, "Blow your mind!"

In the story, Mike and Alisa think they have "Inhibited Sexual Desire" (ISD) symptoms. They are good tantrikas, so they do not have ISD! But they are very busy with work and family. They are not scheduling intimate time.

Thanks to a gifted tantric therapist, Mike and Alisa realize that the Fire Breath is a fantastic technique for them. It works magic, maximizing the results from their precious time together.

Sexual chemistry responds to newness. The couple that tries new things together stays together. There is no rote formula that applies to each individual and every couple. The spirit of adventure itself is the highest aphrodisiac.

Mike and Alisa worked together and found their love solution. Just as the primal Shiva and Shakti, the secret parents of our lives, have accomplished the impossible by giving birth to this magnificent creation we call the universe, the tantric couple who takes their commitment seriously will be able to accomplish anything they set their minds and hearts to do—together.

CHAPTER EIGHT

How to Be Tantric in an Internet World

HOW TO BE TANTRIC IN AN INTERNET WORLD

In Chapter One, I talked about red tantra and white tantra. Red tantra embraces and accepts the body and the senses, sex, and the orgasm, just as they are. Red tantra works with what is—this moment, this life, right now, just as it is. In contrast, white tantra imposes a superstructure of complicated concepts on what is, in essence, the simplest, easiest and most natural action in the world—lovemaking!

The teachings of *Red Hot Tantra* about sex and orgasm originate in the oldest tantra yoga text known, the 4,000-year-old *Vijnana Bhairava*. Its teachings echo around the world.

Vijnana Bhairava means "Divine Consciousness." Much of this sacred text is devoted to the tantric art of fully experiencing the senses. This includes the orgasm. Since it is so old, its 112 techniques are almost certainly remnants of an even older oral tradition. It may be the closest we have to what was taught in the primal tantra of the Divine Mother 6,000 or more years ago.

There are three outstanding versions of *Vijnana Bhairava* available today. For a contemporary tantric perspective, see Osho's lively commentary. Jaideva Singh's translation reflects the views of classic Kashmir Shaivism. Paul Reps telegraphic verses deliver the

Zen punch of a master poet. See Red Hot Resources for more on these books, Internet links, articles, even free downloads of the text.

CELEBRATE THE TANTRIC SECRET OF THE SENSES

As you work with the *Vijnana Bhairava,* keep in mind the way of life in the India of that time. Though the Great Goddess no longer ruled the world, it was still a golden age. The major religions of the world—Christianity, Buddhism, Islam, Judaism—did not yet exist. Their teachings, their commandments, their conflicts, their contradictions were unknown.

You lived locally, in your village, in your forest. There were no electric lights to blot out the thousands of dazzling stars at night. The moon reigned supreme as she sailed across the sky. The only sounds were those of the animals, the insects, the wind rustling the leaves, the liquid music of water flowing in a stream, pulsating in the ocean, falling as rain from the sky against big, waxy palm leaves.

Just imagine if you had been raised in the midst of exquisite natural beauty. It is likely that the solidified, obsessive-compulsive kind of ego that dominates our civilization did not exist back then. Already feeling a near-mystical oneness with nature from birth, it was but one more gentle, joyful step to embrace one of these 112 contemplations and fall with ease into the Unity of Life.

Vijnana Bhairava is the ultimate home-study course in tantra. It is not focused on the tantra of sex, though it reveals its essence. Here is tantra as the art of being truly alive, of celebrating the miracle of the universe by realizing your identity with it. This is tantra as the yoga of beauty and unbroken wholeness. This is a tantra yoga that sees the beauty in everything. This great yoga of surrender to the beauty of the now silences the mind.

Since tantra embraces every level of sincere practice, it is appropriate to use these verses as intentional sensual meditations to open you into the blissful essence of Being. The key is always to enter totally into the momentary dance of sensation. Forget yourself, and in that forgetting, find the Taste of Unity, the Awakening into Wonder, the Bhairava.

Drop the mind. Find the Source that is all at once you, what you are perceiving, and the bridge of perception that bonds you with it. Discover what the tantric sages assert to be the ultimate bliss, the supreme fulfillment—the unity of seer, seeing, and seen.

> **Verse 69:** In sexual orgasm find the delight-filled truth of the Source.
>
> **Verse 70:** Remember and relive the bliss of intimate lovemaking.
>
> **Verse 71:** Contemplate the joy of an experience of intense delight in the moment.

You have already worked with the teachings in Verses 69 and 70. *Red Hot Tantra* is, in essence, an in-depth exploration of them.

NOTICE THE BLISS WITHIN UNCOMMON PLEASURES

Verse 71 refers to situations that don't happen every day. One is meeting a good friend after a long period of separation. Another is the instant in which you experience an unusual rush of pleasure from a unique, meaningful life event.

Your partner has just announced that they won a week-long, all-expenses-paid trip for two to Hawaii—and you're invited! The approach of the *Vijnana Bhairava* is to be alert in the *moment* that this special event happens. If you wait, it's too late. To remember to jump instantly into the gap, the pause induced by your surprise, is difficult!

In this moment, be awake to the spaciousness, to the presence, to the gap. Be alert to this moment-to-moment yoga, the great play of the five senses, the appearance and disappearance of everything within the boundless creativity of Space. Call this Ground of Being anything you like. It is waiting for you.

Look for it when you are in a hot, passionate embrace with the experience. Don't delay. Don't wait to look for that primal Source until you sit on your meditation cushion at your special time or finally manage to get away for that tantric retreat on the beach in

Maui. Be awake today, right now in the midst of the temple of your life. Be aware of the simple, mundane, ordinary, everyday details of daily living. *This* is the teaching of the *Vijnana Bhairava.*

Paradoxically, because Source is everywhere as everything, it is difficult to see. The object, the quickly fading star of the moment, steps in front and says "Look at me!" Now you know, though. The *Vijnana Bhairava* taught you well. Now you know to ask "Yes, my sweet object, you are beautiful, but tell me, where exactly did *you* come from?"

Seize the moment. In that crystal clear instant, there is a throbbing, a pulsation, an expansion from the center of life. Find it, feel it, enter into it, embrace it, merge with it, get lost in it. This cosmic kiss from the Supreme is imprinted on every single sensory experience. Like a friend who wants to be found, but not too easily, the Source of everything is leaving you a trail of breadcrumbs at every turn.

The *Vijnana Bhairava* advises you to go beyond the smooth groove of pleasant flowing sensation by moving even more deeply into it. Look for and melt into the central, pulsing Source of that pleasant sensation *as it is happening.* Otherwise, you went for a ride, but you returned with nothing. Each and every sensation is a collect call from the Source. Take the call. It's for you!

Fortunately, artful practice with pre-planned events works just as well. You don't have to wait for the next big thing. By practicing your personal tantra of opening wide to experiences at home, in a garden, at the beach, and other beautiful, contemplative settings, you develop the habit of alertness to the moment, a skill of effortlessly appreciating the present. As one teacher put it, they call it "the present" because it's a gift!

Embrace the feelings these experiences bring, go into them, become one with them. Trace these sensations to their hidden Source. Leave all concepts behind. Melt into the strong sensations of the moment and fall into the sweet heart of the now. There you will find this amazing one Source, the causeless cause of each and every ecstasy.

As you deepen your embrace of the Real and share its ever-new joy, you will be encouraged to remember the Source more often. An intimacy with life develops that includes your partner and your friends and much, much more. Follow the primordial practices of the *Vijnana Bhairava* and you will make a magnificent new friend—the Universe.

This then is the yoga of the *Vijnana Bhairava*. In every moment, the Source is present. Yet on occasions of strong sensation, the Source takes out an advertisement. Now that you know this secret, you will enjoy these moments even more!

Your tantra may include dressing up in Middle Eastern costumes and dancing to live drumming, naked swims at midnight in the ocean off Maui or making perfect love in romantic, dreamlike settings. It may even involve swinging pujas where sexual fantasies are fulfilled on the spot, which some of my California friends attend!

Tantra does not judge. Tantra says make good use of every situation. Wake up within it! In the totally tantric adventures that are waiting just around the corner for you, you will find many opportunities to enter into the wisdom of Verse 71, the full exploration of uncommon moments of intense delight.

TOTALLY TANTRIC COUPLE'S WEEKENDER KIT

Let's get this party started! I'm going to talk about how to do a local retreat. First, I'll recommend a comprehensive play kit. Then I'll share some fun games and rituals to help make your weekend totally tantric.

In Red Hot Resources, which follows, I share my favorite tantric retreat spots around the world. Don't worry about your budget. If you can afford a good vacation, you can afford these extraordinary hideaways. How does a Mai Tai on a secluded Mayan beach or a tree-house in the jungles of Maui, Hawaii, sound?

I also tell you where to go as a couple to get pampered the tantric way and receive world-class instructions on erotic tantric techniques. Make your tantric dreams come true at these unique retreats.

You need to create a Weekender Kit for your local retreat. Pulling this sweet little package together gets you halfway there. Now you've got a plan and you're in the mood. When you know that you are limited to what you can carry, you quickly discover what you really care about, what *exactly* you must have on hand to have your kind of good time.

If you have certain special games in mind, or you want to go in an S&M direction, then you will need additional toys, tools, and tricks. Still, it's fun to improvise with what's on hand. Did you really think all that free ice from the icemaker down the hall was just for drinks?

Take a deep breath! I'm a Virgo, so the list that follows is comprehensive. I've done my best to cover most situations. I'm assuming there's two of you and that you're on a three-day, two-night, weekend getaway.

Attention! Cell phones and pagers are your enemies! The interruption when it happens is only the beginning. Their invisible tug on your attention throughout the weekend will distract you just when your partner needs you most.

Tantra requires the highest quality of attention. Take care of your affairs before you leave. If you bring your cell phone with you, you must exercise exceptional discipline. Even if you just check your messages, that innocuous first step easily snowballs into more calls, any one of which could be a message that kills your weekend.

How does a busy couple plan a weekend like this?

You know you want it. You know you probably need it! Choose a date together and put in on the calendar. Ink it in just like any other important business or family event.

Make sure your partner knows the exact date. Begin making concrete plans and speaking in terms of specifics. "Either/or" questions have a knack for precipitating a solid response: "Would you like to go to X or to Y?" "Shall we drive or fly?" "Do you want to stay at Tantra Palace again or somewhere new?"

A good rule of thumb is that a happy, busy couple goes out at least one night a week and gets away for a playful holiday at least once every two months. Frankly, if your partner is not willing to commit to special nights and weekends with you, you may have a bigger problem than your hectic schedules!

Even if you can't escape for an entire weekend, get away for Saturday. The morning gives you time to pack and take care of loose ends. Arrive at your hotel between noon and two P.M. on Saturday. Stay the night. Ask for a late checkout on Sunday. Take your time getting back.

When I lived in the Portland area, my partner and I would escape to a tiny beach town on the Oregon coast. The two-hour drive each way was just right. There was a wide beach that was great for long walks, private or together. The town's lack of renown made it perfect for a getaway Even though we were gone only twenty-four hours, we felt refreshed, rejuvenated, and ready for another productive week.

Everyday Basics Weekend Checklist

- ☐ Standard clothes like T-shirts, regular shirts, pants, dressy outfits, underwear
- ☐ Dressy shoes and sandals
- ☐ Deodorant, mouthwash, floss, toothpaste, etc.
- ☐ Brush, comb, hair accessories
- ☐ Lotion, moisturizer, shampoo, conditioner, body wash, sunscreen
- ☐ Perfume, cologne
- ☐ Contact lenses solution and case, extra glasses, supplies for other special needs

Tantric Getaway Checklist

- ☐ Sexy lingerie for her and him (feel free to surprise each other—or give as a gift)
- ☐ Robes—terry or silk
- ☐ Sexy underwear (again, feel free to surprise or be surprised by your partner)
- ☐ Condoms and water-based lubricant (bring extra)
- ☐ Massage oil (more than you think you need—plus the heating and edible varieties)
- ☐ Ostrich feather
- ☐ Silk blindfold or eye mask (red or black)
- ☐ BYOB: Bring Your Own red and amber Bulbs for do-it-yourself boudoir lighting
- ☐ Bubble bath supplies
- ☐ Flavored body butter or frosting
- ☐ Scented or unscented candles and incense
- ☐ Medicine grass for smudging the room (clearing out possible negative energies)
- ☐ Matches
- ☐ Erotic, romantic, sensual CDs (keep six to twelve in their own travel case for different moods)

- ☐ Portable CD boom box (just in case your location doesn't have a working stereo)
- ☐ Erotic videos (if VCR is available)
- ☐ Still camera to record the adventure
- ☐ Video camera (so you can watch yourselves as well as relive your fun later)
- ☐ Sexual stimulants and nutritional support (pharmaceuticals, herbs, vitamins)
- ☐ Chocolate, fruit, favorite foods
- ☐ Favorite drink, such as champagne (non-alcoholic, such as Martinelli's sparkling juices, if engaging in any S&M play)
- ☐ Erotic guides with sexy game ideas
- ☐ Books: *Red-Hot Tantra, The Essential Rumi, Vijnana Bhairava, I Am That*
- ☐ Photocopies of *Red-Hot Tantra* erotic journal page, plenty of pens for writing
- ☐ Drums, rattles, tambourine, hand-held musical instrument(s) of choice
- ☐ Alarm or timer with a soft sound (it goes off, say, four times a day to remind you to be mindful)
- ☐ Tibetan bell with vajra handle to announce the start and end of a ritual or meditation

- ☐ Fresh flowers in a vase (and rose petals for the bed)
- ☐ Sacred items for a temporary altar (statue of a Goddess and a little Buddha or totem, sacred stones, quartz crystals, talisman, holy pictures, silk cloth for the altar surface)
- ☐ Board games, card games or bath games for lovers
- ☐ Vibrators and dildos
- ☐ Nipple clamps (that ice down the hall is nice on nipples, too!)
- ☐ Ping-pong paddle (for serious spanking)
- ☐ Lots of soft cotton rope (for wrist tie-downs—great if you have bedposts—run the rope through a washing machine beforehand to make it soft for your lover)
- ☐ Scissors (for quick release from the tie-down when the knots won't budge)
- ☐ Waterproof sex toys
- ☐ Plenty of extra batteries
- ☐ Sex toy cleaner
- ☐ Pleasure Wipes (for easy clean-up of a hotel room)

TANTRIC GAMES PEOPLE PLAY

Kick off your special weekend with a little ceremony. Light a candle. Read from Rumi, *Vijnana Bjairava* or *I Am That*. Share a poem you wrote that expresses your feelings for each other. Seal it with a kiss, and off you go!

Sometimes getting away creates openness to new experiences. If there is something you've been waiting to ask for, such as a long erotic massage or oral sex from your partner on their knees and blindfolded, this may be the time.

All of *Red Hot Tantra* has been a preparation for your special weekend. Here's your chance to put into practice what you have learned. Leave this book out on the table. Even if your partner has never glanced at it before, they may do so now.

Once again, it is your intention to make this weekend a conscious tantric celebration that makes it one. Before I go out the door on my trip, I bow to the Four Directions and say a prayer to Divine Mother, asking for Her protection and blessings. I will honor Kali, my chosen deity, by repeating "Jai Kali Ma, Jai Kali Ma, Jai Kali Ma." I believe that a simple prayer said with a sincere and grateful heart is the best way to connect with the Higher Power.

Every retreat I go on has a conscious purpose. Each morning of our retreat, I start the day with meditation and reaffirm the purpose of that weekend—whether it's just to have a good time, celebrate my relationship or search within myself for spiritual answers.

Be willing to take personal retreats just for self-healing, too. A two-week retreat by the beach in Encinitas, California, during the early 1980s changed my life. The only structure was a walk on the beach, three great vegetarian meals a day, and the option of counseling from a monk. I had plenty of time for soul-searching.

I was in over my head with some bad people in Hollywood. I had lost my direction in life. I was going down fast! Fourteen days of simple living put me back on track and saved me from actions I might have regretted for many years—if I had lived that long!

I was saved by the clarity of my purpose even when I took a dangerous wrong turn. To get what you want, it helps to know what you want. If you don't know what it looks like, you may not recognize it when it arrives!

Here are ideas for games, rituals, and experiences that are playful, fun, and rewarding. You will find some refreshing twists on some old standards, too:

- **Sacred Space:** What makes a totally tantric weekend different? Yes, you start with the intention, but you need to solidify that intention by making your space sacred. I know people who travel with a portable feng-shui kit when they are staying away from home. It works for them, but I prefer a simple ritual that takes just five minutes. Meditate a few minutes, feeling the energies. Walk around the room, chanting or ringing your Tibetan bell. Smudge the room lightly. Put up your altar. Bow to the Four Directions. Light incense. Place your fresh flowers in a vase. Turn on the music and dance! Take charge of the energies. Hotel rooms have many occupants.
- **The Beach or Mountain Walk:** Okay, you knew about this already. Did you maintain a mind of innocence? Try to feel as if everything is new to you. Even if the surroundings are new, you may be bringing some old issues with you on your walk—anger, bitterness, problems at work, complaints about each other. Even if your weekend environment is spectacular, natural, and fresh, if you carry ugly, stale, old thoughts with you, you've turned your paradise into a garbage dump for your negative thoughts and emotions. Of course, you may need to talk. Just don't forget nature—she's always willing to listen.
- **Soul Gazing:** Get comfortable and face each other. Hold eye contact for several minutes. Feel that you are showing your love and respect through your eyes, reaffirming your connection, honoring your relationship. No need to make this a marathon, but it's a classic. I like to do this in silence. Then each of us says a few words (I want to emphasize "a few"). I think that if you talk too much right after, you lose some of the effect. Soul gazing is a sweet transition into lovemaking. It's a great way to start the day with or without sex. Intimacy has rhythms that need to be honored.

- **One Breath:** Some people teach complex visualizations, imagining a flow of energy between you. They work, but my tantric philosophy is "Less is more." I prefer to sit across from my partner or cuddle and simply let our breaths find their rhythm together, transcending the technique trip. When you're facing each other, it speeds up the process if you lightly hold hands, but even if you don't, your rhythms will find each other and coalesce. This way requires more patience, but you will be blessed with being in the natural, spontaneous flow of life. Now that's One Breath!
- **Word Sandwich:** I learned this from a wild, brilliant, beautiful Tantra teacher who, with his electric-blue eyes and vertical shock of naturally white hair, was perhaps the most striking man I have ever met. I told him that I had a feeling he was from another planet. He smiled and said "Yes, I am. How did you know?" Facing each other, share something positive, then something negative, then something positive again. For example, if you need to share a criticism of your partner, sandwich it between positives like compliments, acknowledgments, and pure, Grade A gratitude. The receiving partner says, "Thank you" after each thought is shared, nothing more. Then switch sides. It may sound contrived, but the Word Sandwich sets up successful communication between people when nothing else is working. If you run into a roadblock with your lovemaking, instead of blaming each other and arguing, try the Word Sandwich. Then you won't have to "eat your words."
- **Fantastic Fantasy:** This is in the "I'll show you mine if you show me yours!" category. Special getaway settings can trigger deeper sharing. Why not tell that fantasy you have been keeping from your partner? I know there's at least one! Here's something to think about: Even if you're fantasy is so outlandish or extreme that your partner prefers to not fulfill it to the letter, you have a very good chance that they will meet you halfway, making your sharing a successful win/win. A shiva asked his shakti if he could have anal sex with her. She said "No, but I'm willing to pretend." They did it doggie style. She

screamed about losing her "anal cherry." The sex was amazing, incredible, the best they ever had. Afterwards, he confessed that he had now lost his fascination with anal sex. This shakti claimed her power. Instead of getting insulted, she negotiated. There are tons of sexual dynamite in your fantasies. It doesn't matter how crazy they are. They're like dreams. Use it to bring you closer together, or lose it.

- **Food Tease:** Another classic that delivers the fun every time! Blindfold your partner. I prefer to surprise them, but you may want them to see what's in store. Reliable sensual choices include flavors of chocolate, sweet liquors like Frangelico, wine, cheese, cherries, grapes. You can introduce citrus fruits now and then to cleanse their palate. As their favorite music is playing, touch a food treat to their lip, on their tongue, so that they take it in their mouth slowly. Take a long time with each item. The point is to tease them. You may think you're torturing them, but when they finally taste it, it will be heavenly due to their anticipation. Notice how you feel, too, for you are enjoying a sensual show. Switch if you like, but this makes a wonderful weekend love gift. The other version, of course, is to feed each other at the same time. Soon it's not just food in your mouths! This game makes a great icebreaker with someone new.

- **Skin Game:** This is about food, too. Take some big, juicy, ripe strawberries. Squeeze the juice on your partner and lick it off. Try honey, yogurt, chocolate syrup, whipped cream, sweet thick liquor, cherry pie filling or chocolate cake icing. (Did you see the movie *9½ Weeks*?)

- **Long Kisses:** No friendly pecks on this trip. Make your kisses long and passionate on purpose. More than words can say, this kind of kiss says, "I'm still in love with you, passionate about you, wanting you." It brings desire boiling to the surface.

- **Surprise Gift:** I've mentioned surprises already, but here I'd like to suggest that you take the time to prepare one very special surprise for your lover. A gift of sexy lingerie or undies is good, but sometimes there is a performance demand implied by erotic gifts. So, do at least one thing that is completely thoughtful, that is only for them. This simple gesture may make your weekend a wonderful memory for years to come. For example, my partner loves to get professional massages. One time when I picked her up, she raved about the massage oil her masseuse was using. My ears perked up. Later that week, I made a special trip to buy some from the masseuse, as it was her proprietary blend. A few months went by. When we went on a tantric weekend getaway, I brought a bottle. She was lying face down on the bed, waiting for her massage, when I applied it to her skin. Instantly, she recognized the unique texture and fragrance of the special oil. Amazed and delighted, she turned herself over, smiled at me, and gave me a long, sweet kiss. She had tears in her eyes. "Now I know you love me," she said. Action is often the best way to say "I love you."

- **Lingerie A-Go-Go:** When you get that gift of sexy underwear or lingerie, put it on. Start the music, dance and let it all go! Nothing says "I love my new lingerie!" like sexy shaking and dancing together.
- **G-Spot Massage:** Not a game, but it can be enormously healing for a woman. At first, it may seem like the man is sacrificing and only the woman is benefiting. Sooner or later, as breakthroughs occur, the blessings rain down on both. Naturally, the relationship is enriched, but there can be a surprising symmetry, so that parallel emotional healings take place within the man as well as the woman. The Muirs in Hawaii popularized this healing experience, which has spread throughout the contemporary tantric community. As they put it, the liquid released during "goddess spot" massage is called "amrita." There are other excellent teachers of a feminist orientation, with all the competence and compassion that implies. There's not enough room here to list them, so check out my suggestions in Red Hot Resources. Since this seemingly

simple technique can bring deep traumas to the surface, if you decide to embrace this process, be willing to stay with it through the weekend, and perhaps well beyond. I learned from books and tapes, but a tantric retreat that features G-spot healing is better, if only because you share in the experiences of other couples, putting it all in perspective. G-spot work may intensify and prolong orgasm, leading to hours of orgasmic ecstasy for some women, but a goal of pure, safe, heartfelt healing is the ideal support for this radical healing journey. Highly recommended *if* you're both ready.

- **Meditate Together:** Another obvious one, but a solid thirty minutes to an hour of complete silence while sitting near each other achieves a synergistic effect not explained by modern science. Tension dissolves, problems are solved, all automatically and without the slightest conscious effort. The majestic silence we sense in vast stretches of nature lives in, and with us, wherever we go. The great sages all point to silence—surely we should listen to them! Sit relaxed and value the mysterious benefit of doing nothing together, even though our modern go-go society cannot imagine a worse fate. Cuddling meditation works sometimes, but sitting nearby and with, instead of lying next to and on, just seems to work better for consciously reaching self-healing spiritual depths.

- **Smell the Roses:** It's so easy to get caught up in a vacation race as you try to get everything in and do it all. Take at least one full hour to be alone and experience the wonders and beauties of nature with your senses. Or try hang-gliding! Yes, it's whatever turns you on right now that gives your life a special sparkle. Think of it as a one-hour tantric meditation mini-retreat. Celebrating the oneness includes looking out for number one! If you don't remember to nurture yourself under ideal conditions far from the demands and distractions of daily life, when will you remember your needs?

It's a Brave New Red Tantric World

THE STRENGTH OF RED TANTRA IS THAT IT EMPHASIZES THE LIVING, beating red-blooded heart of the ancient sexual wisdom that was never lost and will never be lost—the power, glory, ecstasy, and divine revelation that is the conscious sexual climax. In the essence of the orgasm is the answer to all questions, for in That, all questions end. Silence, infinity, light, love, bliss, peace, even if only briefly, reign absolutely.

In that sacred moment beyond time and space, in that organic gap, in that wordless pause of primal pleasure, the supreme truth is revealed. The Great Mother of the Universe lifts up Her skirt and She has no panties. The Secret of Secrets is revealed, the gateway to enlightenment, the Tathagatagarbha—the Womb of the Great Mother of all Buddhas. Yes, ultimate reality is nakedly exposed in total sexual orgasm.

Kali, the great tantric goddess, the queen of sex, the empress of ecstasy, told me so. "I programmed it," She said, "so that any human being can awaken to their true nature through ecstatic sexual surrender! Every orgasm is an opportunity to taste supreme enlightenment!"

Assisted by a loving partner, turned into a powerful meditation through your intention, the sexual orgasm can reveal in a flash the final, blazing truth of your being. Even so, the same ecstatic quest can be accomplished alone, because the truth lives within you, wherever you are and whomever you are with.

Tantra teaches that human beings naturally seek the highest possible pleasure because in the essence of pleasure shines their true nature. In Sanskrit, this pure pleasure at the source of being, which is experienced so vividly at the peak of the sexual orgasm and in the moment of spiritual enlightenment, is known as "ananda," or love-bliss-peace-awareness without limits.

Tantric enlightenment is the art of embodying the Ultimate by being the Intimate. Enlightenment is what you are, and what the world is. Everything is that enlightenment. Recognize it, realize it, relish it, release it. There is nowhere to go but here. There is no time to be here but now. This is it.

When Ram Dass (Richard Alpert) asked his guru about the psychedelic drug LSD, the master smiled and replied "Since Westerners are materialistic, God came to them in the form of a pill."

I humbly submit to you this red tantric view: "We Westerners are obsessed with sex, so God comes to us in the form of the sexual orgasm."

May Divine Mother's blessings rain upon you now as you courageously travel her rich tantric path. May Divine Mother grant you your royal tantric birthright of full bhoga (worldly enjoyment) and full yoga (union with the divine). May Divine Mother give you the Vision of Unity and set you free to be the boundless, loving infinity.

Jai Ma! Jai Ma! Jai Ma!

APPENDIX

Red Hot Resources

RED HOT RESOURCES

DISCLAIMER: The practices, techniques, meditations and other information described in this resource directory are provided for educational purposes only. Please consult your physician for diagnostic and treatment options pertaining to your specific medical condition. Please consult a licensed counselor for assistance with emotional and relationship issues.

The author and publisher of this book are not responsible in any manner whatsoever for any injury, loss or inconvenience which may occur as a result of following instructions herein. It is recommended that before beginning any tantric or similar practice you consult with your physician to determine whether you are medically, physically, and mentally fit to undertake this kind of training.

Are you ready to feast on the fantastic buffet of information about tantra on the Internet? Here are my suggestions, organized chapter by chapter. There are other tremendous resources not mentioned in these seven chapters, so I added a special bonus at the end of these listings called "A Guide to Tantra on the Internet."

If you have positive results with a tantra teacher, sex toy, meditation technique, retreat center or other tantra-related resource, visit my Web site at *www.redhottantra.com* and tell me about it. At my site you will also be able to ask me your tantra questions, subscribe to the free *Red Hot Tantra* e-mail newsletter, download unique, valuable free tantra teachings available nowhere else, get news about my workshops and other teaching activities, and participate in live Internet chat events. Let me know about your wonderful experiences with *Red Hot Tantra* so I can post them on my Web site!

The Internet now competes with television to seduce lovers away from the intimacy they need and deserve. Unlike television, it has made instantly available valuable tantric information, much of it free. Use it!

Many of the suppliers listed under Chapter Eight offer one-stop shopping. Whether you want instructional videos, sensual massage oils or high-tech sex toys, your favorite site may have it all under one roof.

CHAPTER ONE
WHAT IS RED TANTRA?

Actionlove.com teaches Taoist "Level 7" orgasm blending clitoris, G-spot, and cervix. *Healingdao.com* is excellent, with a different approach (Michael Winn).

Erotic dakini poetry: *womensearlyart.net/reference/praise.html*

For a more detailed description of my experience of classic tantric transmission with a dakini (tantric yogini) in Mendocino, CA, see David and Ellen Ramsdale, *Sexual Energy Ecstasy,* Bantam, 1993, pages 201-203. For a parallel experience by a tantric contemporary, see "The Orgasm of Ecstasy" essay about Shri Gurudev Mahendranath's experience of "A Leap into the Cosmos" ("Atma Jyan") with his Shakti: *mahendranath.org/magickpath.mhtml*

For G-spot healing and female ejaculation, see listings for Chapter Seven.

Georg Feuerstein, Ph. D. on "Neo-Tantra": *yrec.org/neotantra.html*

Inside scoop on Adam and Eve: *astradome.com/adam&eve_myth.htm*

Jack Lee Rosenberg, *Total Orgasm,* Random House, 1973. Learn all you need about Reichian and bioenergetic breathwork for maximum orgasm from this great classic. Out of print. *Amazon.com* had 22 copies for sale the day I checked.

Kashmir Shaivism and Buddhist tantra document showing female guru transmitting enlightenment to male disciple in sacred sexual union (see Lady Yeshe Tsogyel): *keithdowman.net/essays/woman.htm* and *khandro.net/dakini_khandro.htm*

Leonard Shlain, *The Alphabet Versus the Goddess,* Viking, 1998. Timeline of change from right brain (nurturing/gathering) to left brain (hunting/killing) as written word replaced images: *alphabetvsgoddess.com*

Lonnie Barbarch, *50 Ways to Please Your Lover: While You Please Yourself,* E. P. Dutton, New York, 1997. All her books are highly recommended.

Merlin Stone, *When God Was a Woman,* New York, Barnes and Noble, 1976. Merlin's message: *pinn.net/~sunshine/whm2000/stone2.html* and *voiceofwomen.com/articles/godwomanart.html*

Miranda Shaw, *Passionate Enlightenment: Women in Tantric Buddhism,* Princeton University Press, 1995. Candid interviews with Miranda: *Enlighteningtimes.com/tantra.htm* and *wie.org/j20/shawintro.asp*

On cervical orgasm pleasure during intercourse, penis size, and best toys for achieving female ejaculation: *holisticwisdom.com/newsletter_6-1-03.htm*

On total surrender, no teacher today is more clear than Ramesh S. Balsekar, successor to Sri Nisargadatta Mahraj: *rameshbalsekar.com, consciousstrikes.org* and *advaita.org* (with Wayne Liquorman). His book *Confusion No More* describes daily life in a natural state of total let-go.

Super Sexual Orgasm by Barbara Keesling, Ph. D. describes spiritual cervical orgasm via "cul-de-sac" intercourse: *audible.com* and *fictionwise.com/ebooks*

Swami Satyananda: *biharyogabharati.net/, yogamag.net/index.shtml* and *tantriccollege.org/what_is_tantra.htm*

Timeless proof of India's ancient erotic wisdom is found in the erotic sculptural art of Konark and Khajuraho: *kamat.com/kalranga/art/sculptures.htm*

To read my personal account of how I became the first person in history to perform an Energy Orgasm for a major television channel, visit *redhottantra.com*

CHAPTER TWO
TANTRIC MEDITATION

A science-based approach to heart meditation: *heartmath.org*

Down-to-earth guidance about the luminous orgasmic mind: *Tibetan Arts of Love,* Gedun Chopel, et al., 1992 and its gay sex variation *Sex, Orgasm and the Mind of Clear Light,* North Atlantic Books, 1998, by noted Tibetan Buddhist Gelukpa scholar Jeffrey Hopkins.

Loving-kindness meditation: *buddhanet.net/metta.htm*

"Mahamudra" or total surrender into orgasmic oneness with the universe (Tilopa's *The Song of Mahamudra*): *keithdowman.net/vajralove/index.htm, kagyu-asia.com* and *lifepositive.com/Spirit/world-religions/Buddhism/tilopa.asp*

Osho's lucid, acclaimed exposition on Tilopa's all-embracing tantric vision is found in *Tantra: The Supreme Understanding: Discourses on the Tantric Way of Tilopa's Song of Mahamudra,* Delhi, Full Circle, 2002, available through

Osho outlets like *oshoviha.org* and *wonderfull-things.com.*

Shiva, Shakti, and Creation: *kheper.net/topics/Tantra/cosmology.html* and *danielodier.com/lalleshwari_e.htm*

Tantra teaches the ego drama of separation has its roots in the relationship with the mother: see Swami Ma, *Mother as First Guru* at *tarayoga.net/mafg.html*

CHAPTER THREE
TANTRIC HEALING

BDSM/spanking basics: *members.aol.com/OldRope/begintip.htm* and *albanypowerexchange.com/BDSMinfo/the_basics.htm*

Entertaining guide with honest reviews of sexual sites: *janesguide.com*

Ever-effervescent Xaviera Hollander has her own Web site: *xaviera.com*

Healing and power through pleasure: *paulagordon.com/shows/resnick*, *hermetic.com/spare/index.htm* and *lifepositive.com/Mind/happiness/pleasure.asp*

Insightful lesbian erotica: *kodiwolf/KWLF/abondageprimer.php*

Khenpo Brothers (Tibetan Buddhist Masters): *padmasambhava.org/pbc*

Kinky learning sites: *kinkycorner.net, gloria-brame.com, blowfish.com, domsublifestyle.com, bondagedirectory.com, alt.com* and *bdsmcafe.com*

Kundalini information and resources: *kundalini-support.com, cit-sakti.com, realization.org/page/topics/kundalini.htm, kundalinicare.com, greatdreams.com/kunda.htm, supernaturalworld.com/chakras.html, lifepositive.com/Spirit/world-religions/hinduism/kundalini.asp, ouroboros.hr/Approach, kundalini-gateway.org* and *savitripriya.org*

My favorite film about the spiritual dimension of sexual surrender "The Story of O": *exxxplicit.com/prods/detailmovie.php?ident=7515*

On the art of simultaneous clitoris and G-spot stimulation, see David and Ellen Ramsdale, *Sexual Energy Ecstasy,* Bantam, 1993, pages 187-191.

Tantra yoga practices and perspective on anal muscle mastery: *Asana, Pranayama, Mudra, Bandha,* by Swami Satyananda (see sites in Chapter One).

Tantric S&M: *sensuoussadie.com/spiritualityquotes, spiralway.com/mcybelle/interviews.htm, domin8rex.com,* and *yourkey.sufferware.com/sc.htm*

"The Sexual Life of Children": *home.wanadoo.nl/martinson/index.html*

This sex chakra healing meditation was inspired by a workshop taken with bioenergy healer Mietek Wirkus (Bio-Relax, Bethesda, MD): *mietekwirkus.com*

CHAPTER FOUR
TANTRIC TOUCHING

Clothespin nipple play: *gmsma.cog/newslink/titplay.html, steelskys.com/clips.htm* and *stockroom.com/sec03.htm*

Conventional but comprehensive: *eroticguide.com/toys/toys/lubes.html*

Erotic massage (hands-on manuals): *sexuality.org/erotmass.html* and *them.ws/frontpage/?page=massage* (insights into seductive massage).

ESO: How You and Your Lover Can Give Each Other Hours of Extended Sexual Orgasm, Alan P. Brauer, Donna J. Brauer, Warner Books, 1989, is the source book for the manual stimulation-style of expanding the orgasm.

Eye-opening discussion of lubricants and their effects (including the "Albolene" recommended by the Brauers): *joanelloyd.com/fbesolube.htm*

Goddesses: *pathofthemother.com, mothergoddess.com* and *srividya.org*

Group massage scene: *libchrist.com/newsletter/Spring97.html*

Hindu Divine Mother:
sivanandadlshq.org/download/godmother.htm

Homemade massage oil recipe: thirty drops of essential oil for every one ounce of carrier oil (almond and jojoba oil blend).

Patricia Taylor, Ph.D.'s in-depth exploration:
expanded-orgasm.com

Quality masks and blindfolds: *drugstore.com, frankbush.com, mypleasure.com,* etc. Note: Prices vary, so shop around!

Tantric Yoga and the Wisdom Goddesses, David Frawley, Lotus, 2000.

CHAPTER FIVE
TANTRIC SEEING

Astral (OBE) sex and travel: *realmagick.com/articles/53/853.html* (Robert Bruce), *astralpulse.com, robertpeterson.org* and *williambuhlman.com*

Calling Kali: *exoticindiaart.com/article/Kali, yoni.com/bitch/Kali.shtml, liberalmafia.org/darkgoddesses/Kali.html, goddessworld.com/darkone.html, altered-states.net/tantrahome/Kali/index.htm, sivasakti.com/local/art-kali.html, geocities.com/SoHo/Lofts/2938/linkspagn3.html, calcuttaweb.com/religious.htm, kalimandir.org* (Kali temple in Laguna Beach, CA) and *spiritofmaat.com*

Carlos Castaneda Style Shamanic Dreaming: *Castaneda.com, uazone.org/naph/ccarlos/ccarloslinks.html, webreathe.com/truemind* and *magicalblend.com/library/readingroom/articles/dreaming.html*

Conscious dreaming groundwork: *soulfuture.com, dreamgate.com, dr-dream.com, tryskelion.com/dreamakr.htm, henryreed.com, lifepositive.com/mind/paranormal/dreams/dream-reality.asp, lifetreks.com/lifetreks2/incubation.asp, ingom.dimensiondancers.de/en/text/dreamland/index.html,* and *creativespirit.net/henryreed/dreamquest/incubation.htm*

Dream journal:
soulfuture.com/dreams/phase2_dream_symbols.asp, mentalhelp.net/psyhelp/chap15/chap15g.htm and *WritingTheJourney.com*

Dream magic:
angelfire.com/realm2/amethystbt/dreammagick6.html and *wisdomsdoor.com*

Dream Supplements: *cures-not-wars.org/mdreams.html (melatonin), mazatecgarden.com* (source for Calea zacatechichi, Mexican Dream Herb)

Encountering Kali: In the Margins, at the Center, in the West, Rachel Fell McDermott, Ed., Jeffrey J. Kripal, Ed., University of California Press, 2003.

Essential clove oil (and other oils) source: *aromaticessentials.com*

Garfield interviews: *sawka.com/spiritwatch/patricia_garfield.htm* and *intuition.org/txt/garfield.htm* (Mishlove *Thinking Allowed* transcript)

I Am That, Nisargadatta Maharaj, Chetana Press, Bombay, 1992. On this realized master (d. 1981) of Tantric Nath lineage started by legendary Dattatreya: *nisargadatta.net, advaita.org, nonduality.com, realization.org* and *prahlad.org*

Linda Magallon, *Mutual Dreaming: When Two or More People Share the Same Dream,* Pocket Books, 1997. Linda Magallon offers "Basic Skills for Mutual Dreaming" at *members.aol.com/dreampsi/archive/mutualdream1.html*

Lucid dreaming audio support: "Lucid Dreaming" (four Hemi-Sync® tapes), *probablefuture.com* (theta/delta mind entrainment empowerment CD)

Lucid dreamwork: *dreamweb.ch/don/, dteck.chalmers.se/~d4carlos/lucid, dreams.ca/lucid.htm* and *eliasforum.org/library/lucid_dreaming_overview.html*

Patricia Garfield, Ph. D., *Pathway to Ecstasy: the Way of the Dream Mandala, Creative Dreaming, Your Child's Dreams* at *patriciagarfield.com*

Robert Monroe, *Journeys Out of the Body,* Main Street Books, 1973.

Stephen LaBerge, Lucidity Institute and NovaDreamer: *lucidity.com*

The Gospel of Sri Ramakrishna, transl. Swami Nikhilananda, The Ramakrishna-Vivekananda Center of New York, 1977. The unabridged version.

The most poetic translation of *The Bhagavad Gita* is by Stephen Mitchell. *Gita4free.com* and *bhagavadgitausa.com* offer excellent free versions online.

Tibetan Dream Methods: Tenzin Wangyal Rinpoche, *The Tibetan Yogas of Dream and Sleep,* Snow Lion, Ithaca, New York, 1998, at *ligmincha.org*

Yoga nidra waking dream meditation (guided tantric meditation on CD or tape for entering theta and delta states): *scand-yoga.org* and *swamij.com*

CHAPTER SIX
TANTRIC HEARING

Discover Your Personal Visual, Auditory, Kinesthetic Pattern: *lifepositive.com/mind/personal-growth/nlp/nlp-effect.asp*

Enneagram role-play alternative: *enneamotion.com, ninepoints.com, 9waysofworking.com, authenticenneagram.com* and *ideodynamic.com*

Journaling resources: *geocities.com/HotSprings/Spa/5114/journal.htm, writersdigest.com/articles/fill_page_one.asp, geocities.com/paintedtile, the-intuitive-self.com, selfhelpmagazine.com/articles/health/journal.html, lifepositive.com/Mind/personal-growth/write-therapy/write.asp, inspiredtojournal.com, geocities.com/Athens/Acropolis/7086/selfhelp.html new.blogger.com/home.pyra* and *writingthejourney.com*

Spiritual music resources: *smcmarin.com/yogashoppe.htm, tantricshamanism.com, tantramag.com/play.html, bhagavandas.com, firedance.org/chants, krishnadas.com* and *fourgates.com/musicdevotion.asp*

CHAPTER SEVEN
TANTRIC BREATHING

A handy summary of the Five Tibetans (Mi Zong exercises) and a quick guide to books on the five rites can be found at *shapeshift.net/5tibetans*. Here is a secret oral teaching from a Russian master: When you are instructed to tense all of your muscles at once, pull up firmly at the anus and perineum, too. This increases the flow of life energy from the root chakra, improving health and vitality.

All about kriyas: *kundalini-gateway.org/polls/po_kriya.html* and *kundalini-teacher.com/symptoms/kriyas.html*

For practical help with Energy Orgasm, visit *redhottantra.com* Reichian style differences can be confusing. The works of Alexander Lowen, John Pierrakos and Jack Rosenberg are reliable and objective.

Glenn H. Mullin, *Tsonghkapa's Six Yogas of Naropa*, Snow Lion, 1997 is a remarkable guide to the body's energy channels (with parallels to Taoist yoga).

Hatha yoga "uddiyana bandha": *yrec.org/bandha.html* and *rainbowbody.com/asana/bandha.htm#Uddiyanabandha*

Harley Swiftdeer Reagan Metis Medicine Society (training in "Chuluaqui Quodoushka" or Cherokee energy orgasm technique): *deertribe.com*

"How to Have Energy Orgasms" by Annie Sprinkle with Jwala (article based on the Cherokee method): *rahoorkhuit.net/library/yoga/tantra*

ISD (Inhibited Sexual Desire): *psychotherapist.net/sextherapy/isd.htm* and *mothernature.com/Library/bookshelf/Books/62/54.cfm*

Jack Johnston, M.A. can be reached at *multiples.com*

Kundalini information and resources: *kundalini-support.com, cit-sakti.com, realization.org/page/topics/kundalini.htm, kundalinicare.com, greatdreams.com/kunda.htm, supernaturalworld.com/chakras.html, lifepositive.com/Spirit/world-religions/hinduism/kundalini.asp, ouroboros.hr/Approach and savitripriya.org*

Lama Thubten Yeshe, *The Bliss of Inner Fire: Heart Practice of the Six Yogas of Naropa*, Wisdom Publications, Boston, 1998. *Lamayeshe.com* is official site. Hans Taeger recalls the kundalini master's warm personality at *iol.ie/~taeger*

Merilyn Tunneshende Toltec energy orgasm: *uazu.net/notes/merilyn.html*

"Sex is not what you think. Sex is natural LSD." David and Ellen Ramsdale, *Sexual Energy Ecstasy*, Bantam, 1993, page 363. Working individually with the self-empowerment meditation in "Orange Light of Joy" may enhance your Cosmic Fire Breath embrace.

To better understand experiences of unity achieved by doing the Energy Orgasm, the Fire Breath and other tantric techniques, see Vedantic "I Am That" insight (also called Advaita Bhavana or "Universal Love for All as One's Self"): *realization.org/page/topics/advaita_Vedanta.htm, gangaji.org, sv.uit.no/student/dinteo/ibooks.html, nondual.com/links.html, tantriccollege.org/KSTArticle.htm, anandashram.org* and *sentient.org*

Yab-Yum God/Goddess position: *mandalas.com/tantraeyes.htm, oztantra.com/b_magazine.html* and *exoticindiaart.com/article/tantra*

Yogi Bhajan Breath of Fire: *geocities.com/cartboy_2000/kundalini.html, kundaliniyoga.org/pranayam.html* and *kundaliniyoga.homestead.com/tantra.html*

CHAPTER EIGHT

HOW TO BE TANTRIC IN AN INTERNET WORLD

A respected, highly readable scholarly translation of *Vijnana Bhairava* made in consultation with Swami Lakshman Joo: Jaideva Singh, *The Yoga of Delight, Wonder, and Astonishment,* State University of New York Press, 1991.

Coleman Barks, *The Essential Rumi,* HarperCollins, New York, 1995.

Drumming: *myshamanicvision.com, earthdrum.com, ubdrumcircles.com, animana.org/tab3/31_INTRO.shtml, ritualdrum.col, drums.org, drumcafe.co.za, jimdonovanmusic.com, unclemafufo.com, layneredmond.com, carlmccolman.com*

Eagle's Nest wooded romantic getaway (Inverness, California): *blackthorneinn.com*

Female ejaculation (books/videos): *LawlessSpirit.com, fatalemedia.com, doctorg.com, houseochicks.com, tantraattahoe.com, wetfemaleejaculation.com, thegspotvideo.com, orgasmaniacs.com/books.shtml* and *anniesprinkle.org*

Find all those toys and supplies, from bubble bath and sexy games to heating and edible massage oils to weekend play kits to waterproof vibrators and Ylang-Ylang scented candles, at these reliable sources. Browsing these mostly woman-owned retail sites is a fantastic way to find out what's available. Ideas abound to help you create personalized play scenes and do-it-yourself weekender kits (inspired by their pricey prepackaged offerings!). And check out the free, informative how-to articles: *goodvibes.com, mypleasure.com, babeland.com, drugstore.com, kleptomaniac.com, girlsliketoparty.com, LawlessSpirit.com, libida.com, kittenstoyroom.com, sexy-jewelry.com, condom.com, houseochicks.com, tantra.com* and *tantra-sex.com*

Free downloads of *Vijnana Bhairava Tantra:* *lorinroche.com/1.htm, danielodier.com/vijnana_e.html, sivasakti.com/local/osho/vijnana-bhairava-tantra-vol1/index.html* and *shivashakti.com/vijnan.htm*

G-spot healing: *sourcetantra.com, aloha.net/~alessin/LoveLady.html* (step-by-step instructions) and *womensexualitycenter.com*

Getaway to Posada Dos Ceibas, eight circular beachfront bungalows, near Mayan ruins, south of Tulum, Mexico, on the Caribbean coast: *dosceibas.com*

How to put together an S&M play kit (and much more): *sexuality.org*

I Am That by Nisargadatta Maharaj. Acclaimed modern spiritual classic.

In his bestseller *The Power of Now,* deservedly popular Eckhart Tolle echoes the 4,000 year-old *Vijnana Bhairava* message: *eckharttolle.com*

Jan's guide to everything you need to create a beautiful tantric love nest (exotic wall hangings, pillows, candles, incense): *tantricjoy.com/resources.html*

Maya Tulum getaway, low-key, romantically rustic retreat and resort, a yogi favorite, south of Tulum, Mexico, and near Mayan ruins: *mayatulum.com*

Neem Karoli Baba (Mahraj Ji): *neemkarolibaba.com/home108.html*

Nudist/naturist getaway (near Cancun, Mexico): *caribbeanreefclub.com*

Osho provides his original commentary and answers questions on the 112 meditation techniques of the *Vijnana Bhairava (Vigyan Bhairav)* Tantra in the 1184 page, one-volume edition, *The Book of Secrets,* St. Martin's Press, New York, 1998. Nicely complementing this masterpiece are Osho's elegant insights in two volumes into the Royal Song of Saraha, *The Tantra Experience* and *Tantric Transformation.* Saraha has been called "the Founder of [modern] Tantra." Fourth in

Osho's quartet of in-depth commentaries on tantra's greatest classics is *Tantra: The Supreme Understanding,* a liberating view into Tilopa's Song of Mahamudra.

Paul Reps, *Zen Flesh, Zen Bones,* Tuttle, 1957, 1998. "Centering" section is poet Reps succinct, lyrical version. He studied with Swami Joo.

Personalized tantric retreats for couples by tantra teacher couples: *oceanictantra.com* (private sessions with Kutira and Raphael in Maui paradise); *ecstaticliving.com/AmritaSprings.htm* (Steve and Lokita's B&B casita with tantra coaching for couples two hours north of San Francisco), and *tantra-sex.com* ("Couples Weekend" in Ontario "Love Nest" with Pala Copeland and Al Link).

Ram Dass, *Be Here Now* author: *ramdasstapes.org* and *ramdass.org*

Sage Sri Ramana Maharshi embodied the Wisdom of Silence: *ramana-maharshi.org* (offers free e-book downloads) and *arunachala.org*

Secluded rainforest lodge getaway in Costa Rica: *lunalodge.com*

Sensual trance dance music: *mymastermusic.com/links.html, rafadelic.com/links.htm, danceparadise.curvedspaces.com/dp-001.htm, ecstaticspirit.com/Bistro/dancecds.html, backroadsmusic.com, heartmagic.com, doctorg.com/sensual_music.htm, precioustantra.com* and *kikos.com/debcriss*

Smudging (space clearing): *sundancersage.homestead.com/smudge.html, nativecircle.com/HERBS.htm* and *spirit-bears-tipi.50megs.com/sage.html*

Spiritual retreats: *expandinglight.org, women-traveling.com, womens-spiritual-retreats.com, tantricshamanism.com, retreat-co.co.uk, breitenbush.com/html/retreats.html, esalen.org, retreatsforhealing.com, interluderetreat.com/links.htm, dhamma.org, spiritrock.org, dharma.org*

Swami Lakshman Joo, Kashmir Shaivism and Lord Shiva: *kousa.org, ksf.org, exoticindiaart.com/article/shivalinga, tantriccollege.org/KSTArticle.htm* and *dlshq.org/download/lordsiva.htm*

Tantric honeymoon planning: *doctorg.com/romantic_travel.htm* and *honeymoons.miningco.com/cs/tantricsex/index.htm*

Ten Zen Ox: *santosha.com/philosophy/oxherdingpictures_1.html*

Tibetan hand bells (space clearing): *tibetantraditions.com, khandro.net, pilgrimshandicrafts.com* and *tibetshop.com*

Top tantric week-long vacation retreat: *sourcetantra.com* (Seminars in Maui, Hawaii, with Charles and Carolyn Muir consistently get great reviews.)

Tree House Cottage (and more) getaway in Hana, Maui, Hawaii: *hanahale.com*

A GUIDE TO TANTRA ON THE INTERNET

In this listing, the first site is not better than the twelfth. All offer unique value. Several of these sites simply do not show up in conventional searches. Here are my picks for the top twelve tantric Web sites, followed by other useful sites:

1. *tantra.org:* Good reliable overview of Western tantra today.
2. *shivashakti.com:* Mike Magee. Huge collection of tantric texts.
3. *tantraworks.com:* Nik Douglas (co-author of *Sexual Secrets*).
4. *LawlessSpirit.com:* Therapist Lisa Lawless' free artistic female ejaculation movie clips alone are worth the visit. Informative free newsletter and honest, useful insights from "Make Your Own Dildo Kits" to "Sexual Mindfulness." Thought provoking.
5. *alchemicaltaoism.com:* Unique treasure of free Taoist sexual alchemy knowledge. Deep, precise insider cultivation secrets.

6. *mumyouan.com/i/ae-i.html:* Eighty playful, practical Zen Tantra pages from renegade Zen Master EO on finding ego-death and nothingness (no-mind) in total orgasm. Houzan Suzuki (Mumyouan) translated the late EO's manual for us.
7. *domin8rex.com:* Mystress Angelique Serpent. Shakti sage skillfully blends kundalini, tantra, S&M, enlightenment. Extensive free video. You are guaranteed to learn something!
8. *anniesprinkle.org:* Tantric pioneer, erotic priestess, transcendental porn star, body art entertainer, cosmic cheerleader. Annie's work helps us all be free. Visit this site!
9. *actionlove.com:* Hot loving Taoist sex for today. G-spot/ cervical orgasm insights. Information-packed answers to many sex questions. Balances traditional tao sex teachings.
10. *luckymojo.com/sacredsex.html:* A historical tour of European and American occult tantric sex experiments.
11. *sivasakti.com:* A unique site! Sensitive, insightful.
12. *redhottantra.com:* Hey, I couldn't leave myself out!

Alternative community: *firedance.org* and *mcbridemagic.com*

AOL Tantric forum: *members.aol.com/tantric4um/forumlog.html*

Belly dancing music and instruction: *visionarydance.com, nevina.com, AliahsCloset.com, belly-dancing-bellydance.com, desertmoondance.com, bellydancingbyzamoras.com* and *bellydancingvideos.com*

Contemporary yoga: *layogamagazine.com, yogadirectory.com, spiritofyoga.com.au/links.htm, yogajournal.com, santosha.com, yogasuperstore.com, yogafinder.com, rainbowbody.net, scand-yoga.org, movingintostillness.com* and *globalfriendsnet.com/links/yogameditation.html*
Yes, yoga is good for sex, as this video shows: *bettersexthroughyoga.com*

Creative sex education: *houseochicks.com/vulvauniversity, sexualpositionsfree.com, abbys-sexual-health.com, jackinworld.com, sexuality.org, masterejaculation.com* and *liarmag.com/tantra_sex.html,*

"Divine Sexuality" essay by author: *tantra.com/divine.html, tantra-sex.com/tantra-articles.html* and *dorje.com/8080/netstuff/dharma/buddha10*

European pharmaceutical enhancement of sex and brain function: *qhi.co.uk, smart-drugs.com, nootroopics.com* and *nubrain.com*

Female orgasm insights: *purpletights.com/sex/gspot.htm, healthtao.com, clitoris-information.com, evesgarden.com/Drpatti/archive/index.html, after-glow.com/femclitorg.html, clitical.com, anniesprinkle.org* and *bettydodson.com*

First choice for gay and bisexual tantra instruction: *bodyelectric.org*

Hindu spirituality links: *sabarimalathanthri.com/html/hindusource.htm*

Insights from Jonn Mumford, *Ecstasy Through Tantra*, Llewellyn, 1988: *llewellynjournal.com/article/360* and *omplace.com/articles/Tantra_Interview.html*

Jack Johnston's multiple orgasm "Key Sound" technique for men and women works! Jack offers chats and great support, too: *multiples.com*

Lee Lozowick, *The Alchemy of Love and Sex,* Hohm Press, 1995, is an honest reality check for every tantrika: *leelozowick.com* and *hohmpress.com*

Modern male tantra masters: *barrylong.org* and *deida.com* (David Deida)

Osho's legacy is a thriving global community of consciousness celebrating the cosmic heart unity of sex, love, surrender, tantra, ego-loss, and enlightenment: *oshoworld.com, oshoviha.org, otoons.com, osho.com, sannyasnews.com, sannyas.net, sannyasworld.com, sannyas.org, dolano.com, ishwara.com, oshana.org, living-dying.com, osholeela.co.uk, livingsatsang.nl, humaniversity.nl, oshouta.de, oshorisk.dk, meditationfrance.com, mevlana-community.com, Barnett.sk/software/sos/osho/osho-talks, osho.co.uk, rupda.com, samdarshi.com, globalserve.net/~sarlo/Ratings.htm, fortunecity.com/marina/tidal/2339/, newagegossip.co.uk, tyohar.com, croydonhall.co.uk* and *connection-medien.de*

Sex and spirituality: *members/tripod.com/~maenad/sensual1/html* and *lifepositive.com/Body/sexuality/sex-spirituality.asp*

Sincere, helpful, informative tantric and taoist sex and yoga sites: *tantrapm.com, jonnmumfordconsult.com, tantriccollege.org, tantricspirit.com, tantra.com, sacredtantra.com, oztantra.com, tantricshamanism.com, healingdao.com, precioustantra.com, rahoorkhuit.net/library/yoga/tantra, tantramag.com, tantra-sex.com, umaatantra.com, schooloftantra.com, 1tantra.com, hai.org, swami-center.org, ojai.net/raymondpowers/INDEX.HTM, yogaesoteric.net, geocities.com/HotSprings/Villa/4480/index.htm, 3mmagic.com, tantramagazine.com, bogomudr.org/eng/main/, ecstaticliving.com, sacredsexyes.com, taomagic.com, tantrika.com, home.sprynet.com/~ttribe/, tantricyoga.net, geocities.com/iona_m/Virtualtantra/ball-lightning.html, sacredmountainretreat.org, martinj.dircon.co.ukjadegardentantra.com, tantralaboratory.com, goddessherself.com, tantraattahoe.com, tantrabliss.com*

Spiritual orgasm spectrum: *universal-tao.com/article/quest.html, ladyfire.com/hits_421.htm* and *silentground.com/VisionaryAlchemy.htm*

Tantra links: *martinj.dircon.co.uk/page7.html, phs2.net/cwi/L3/o795li.htm, martinmyst.net/tantra.html, dmoz.org/Society/Sexuality/Tantra/Workshops/, kheper.net/topics/Tantra/links.htm, tantra-sex.com/tantra-links.html, tantraworks.com/twlinks.html* and *spiritualskyincense.com/love-links.htm*

Tantra, tao, magick sex books: *anathemabooks.com/sex_magick.shtml, used.addall.com* (free used book search), *amazon.com* (out of print books).

Tantric couple rejuvenation: *yogajournal.com/wisdom/450.cfm, yogajournal.com/wisdom/463.cfm, lifepositive.com/Body/sexuality/sex-energize.asp, llewellynjournal.com/article/388, sourcetantra.com/media-reviews/yoga-journal.htm, tantra-sex.com/tantra-article3.html, myria.com* and *bostonphoenix.com/archive/features/98/01/15/TANTRIC_SEX .html*

Tantric escorts and massage (including G-spot healing): *orient.ro, cosmic-tantra.ch, goddesstemple.com, everlastingtouch.com* and *whitelotuseast.com*

Tantric orgasm sex magic: *greendome.org/archives/tantra/tantra.html* and *geocities.com/HotSprings/Villa/4480/magick.htm*

Tantric texts translated by Sir John Woodroffe: *sacred-texts.com/tantra/maha/index.htm, sacred-texts.com/tantra/sas/index.htm*

Tantric "weightless" lovemaking for couples, back relief: *loveswing.com*

Ultimate in high-tech sex for women, men, and couples: *sybian.com*

Whole brain sex and orgasm: *hometown.aol.com/discord23/gen.htm, viewzone.com/amygdala/* and *h2net.net/p/nslade/Papers/sex.html*

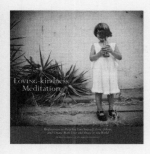

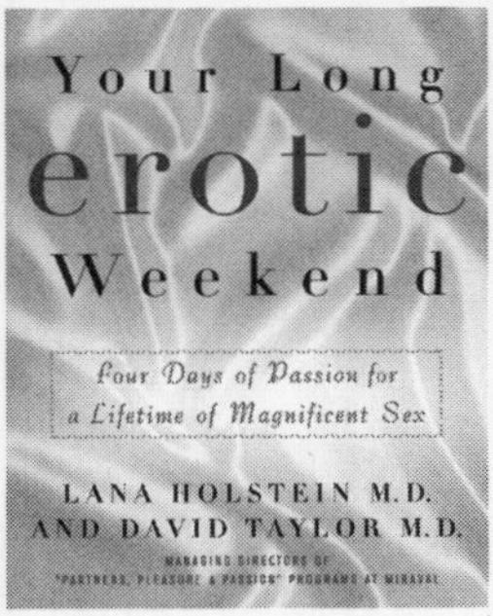

YOUR LONG EROTIC WEEKEND

By Lana Holstein, MD and David Taylor, MD

ISBN: 1-59233-061-4

$22.00/$12.99

Hardcover; 240 pages

Available wherever books are sold

You're just a weekend away from sexual bliss!

You don't have to pay thousands of dollars for one of those fabulous sexuality workshops at a world-class resort that are all the rage nowadays. *Your Long Erotic Weekend* is a workshop in a book—written by the very creators of the Canyon Ranch and Miraval sex workshops, Drs. Lana Holstein and David Taylor. This dynamic husband and wife team takes you step-by-step on a passionate journey of self-exploration:

Day One: You and your lover rekindle that spark, learning to tune into each other's sexual energy.

Day Two: He pleases her—and unleashes her inner sex goddess.

Day Three: She returns the favor for her warrior lover—and pleases him as he's never been pleased before.

Day Four: The two of you become one in a mind-altering, soul-shattering ecstatic union that rocks your world forever.

With *Your Long Erotic Weekend* you're not in sexual dullsville anymore. You'll learn how to awaken your sensual selves, rekindle that sexual spark, master the Tantric secrets of orgasm, and take one another to heights of passion you've only dreamed about. This is sex like you've never had before!

About the Authors

Lana L. Holstein, MD and David J. Taylor, MD, have been married for 28 years. Together they created the Canyon Ranch sex workshops and currently run a four-day retreat at Miraval, one of the world's premier spas. Holstein is the author of *How to Have Magnificent Sex* (Harmony) and the companion video, which is currently featured on PBS in fundraisers across the country.